Rise of the
Magpies

Rise of the Magpies

Newcastle United's Renaissance

Abi Smith

pitch

First published by Pitch Publishing, 2024

Pitch Publishing
9 Donnington Park,
85 Birdham Road,
Chichester, West Sussex,
PO20 7AJ
www.pitchpublishing.co.uk
info@pitchpublishing.co.uk

A CIP catalogue record is available for this book from the British Library.

ISBN 978 1 80150 763 9

MIX
Paper | Supporting responsible forestry
FSC® C013604

Printed and bound in the UK on FSC® certified paper in line with our continuing commitment to ethical business practices, sustainability and the environment.

Typesetting and origination by Pitch Publishing

Printed and bound by CPI Anthony Rowe, UK

Contents

To the old and the new Magpies …

Grampy, Chris, Lily, Henry and Tommy.

Acknowledgements

MY FIRST line of thanks must go to Pitch Publishing for agreeing that a book about the mighty Toon was indeed worth commissioning – and for working with me (boxing, tennis and now football writer) once again.

Thanks to everyone who gave me their thoughts and opinions of NUFC over the past year: for answering messages, emails, social media threads, texts about a whole range of questions I had that spanned decades of the club's history and always with an 'it's no bother' or 'happy to help' reply. Thank you to all in the Toon Army who chatted away to Henry, to me, to my husband, Chris, when we were in Newcastle, and thanks to the students who showed me that the Magpie contingent held strong here in the south when I needed confirmation of speculation, of theories and ideas. You'll read many quotes in here that simply have just a name linked to them, from the many fans I've met and chatted to who didn't always give me surnames or titles and didn't need to offer me anything more than their valuable insights.

Massive thanks to Rob for always answering my messages and agreeing to be my go-to, and also for giving Henry the opportunity to experience his first Newcastle home game. To Alan and Sharon for sending me insights and helpful background knowledge, and to Callum, Isaac and Geordie Josh for giving me your views during science lessons and in the corridors and over IG.

My biggest thanks goes to Grampy, without whom I wouldn't have even entertained this idea. You're always my biggest supporter and I love you for that. As is your son, whom I love too, of course.

And to Lily, Henry and Tommy. Bob, this book has always and will always be for you. Tomski, if you sleep in your own bed, I'll read you a chapter of this every night. Lils, you're simply the best – and not just because you're the first born into the new generation of Toon Army supporters without realising it.

Anecdotally, I also spend a lot of time in a secondary school where football supporters are vast, varied and very vocal, and I frequently get asked the age-old question: 'Who do you support, Miss?' My answer, every time, is simply: 'The best team in the world.'

Prologue

MY LINKS with Newcastle are, at best, minimal. Full disclosure. I love Cheryl Cole but I didn't love the sip of Newcastle Brown Ale I once tried. I religiously watched *Geordie Racer* as a child and Ant and Dec's PJ and Duncan's song was the theme tune to my teenage years. I was always 'ready to rumble'. I have two magpies that visit my garden on a regular basis and who have even taken up residence in the willow tree at the end of the lawn, which I believe signifies a seal of approval from the Magpies in general. Living in a leafy Sussex village meant that the local pubs were awash with the red, blue and white shirts of the Gunners, the Red Devils, the Blues and Pensioners, and Spurs every time I fancied a quiet drink.

No mighty Magpies to speak of, yet here I am finding myself writing about one of the greatest, if not *the* greatest, teams in the world and I have goosebumps at the thought of such a privilege – perhaps because this will earn major mum points when it comes to my sons Henry and Tommy, who worship the black-and-white ground that Newcastle United play on, yet have only visited St James' Park on two occasions (Why can't we move to Newcastle, Mum? I can get a job in the Labour Club.). Asking your son which football team he supports largely depends on the intensity of the previous generation – the pressure from the top. But it can be formed and then nurtured all by its own accord and on its own merit.

My father-in-law's family originated from the north of England and found their way south by way of his mother, who was born six miles from St James' Park, in Jarrow. Jennifer Peters, or Jen as she was known, left Newcastle before the start of the Second World War, as many did, to find work further south. Her father was one of the many men who took part in the Jarrow Crusade, the protest march against mass unemployment in the town. Palmer's shipyard, the largest employer in Jarrow, had closed due to the Great Depression, leaving over 70 per cent of the town unemployed. Jen's father joined around 200 other men on the march from Jarrow on 5 October 1936 to deliver a petition from the people of the town to the House of Commons. This crusade took them 26 days and became a defining moment of the 1930s. Jen left Jarrow, all she knew and loved, her family and her roots and moved to Aylesbury, in the heart of Buckinghamshire (coincidentally the same county in which a future Mr Edward Howe was born), to work in a hat factory. It was there she met Christopher Smith, got married and had four children, but her allegiance, love and admiration to her hometown and the club that shadowed her childhood was passed down to her son, grandson and (not that she'd know it, sadly) her great-grandsons.

Holding firm to his northern roots amid the sea of London clubs and southern seaside teams that flooded the pubs and social clubs, my father-in-law felt, at times, a lone cheering voice of the black-and-white army in the south. When his son and, later, grandsons were old enough, of course the membership increased. Although being careful not to push his football allegiance on to them, it formed naturally while watching the likes of Peter Beardsley, Barry Venison, Rob Lee, Lee Clark and then later Dan Burn, Kieran Trippier and Nick Pope.

Which goes to the heart of this book. My connection, although from afar, is as strong as those that grew up in the shadow of St James' Park and celebrate a win with a pint in The Strawberry. My father-in-law's passion for a club, then my husband and then my sons, a three-generational passion that defies geography but defines their relationship. My own connection with the club has over the years, ranged from a distant interest: 'Sorry they lost babe, what do you want for your tea?' – to seeing Babygros online and thinking that baby Henry will look so cute in in the black and white stripes. I even bought a share in the club in 2006 as a pre-wedding present for my husband-to-be. I framed the certificate and it's up on my study wall ... wonder if it's worth anything now? And can I legitimately – as much as the gifting website giving authenticity allows – call myself a shareholder? I might try.

What I lack in knowledge of NUFC I've gained through hours of research and interviews with those kind enough to tell me – in animated passion – every detail I should need. What I lack in player facts, stats and figures I've gained through hours of listening to Henry most evenings. His knowledge of the club has been part of his life for just 11 short years but is seemingly seeped in the history of his ancestors.

'Every time I go to my room I listen to 'Blaydon Races' and 'Local Hero' to re-enact my time in Newcastle,' he tells me.

A book on a football team is only as good as the authentic voice that tells it, so, firstly, while my apology at the beginning of this still stands, my insight into a club that has such warmth, passion, enthusiasm and pride has infiltrated my bones and will hopefully show in the black words on the white pages. If there's one thing I've learned about writing this book, it's that the hearts and souls of the people of Newcastle seep out from the grass of St James' Park and infiltrate those showing willing and wanting to be accepted.

A fan, by definition, is a term sometimes used interchangeably with a football supporter, but most people believe there's a distinction between the two. If we're speaking in general terms, a 'fan' is someone who, according to some, has a casual interest in a sport and potentially a specific team, whereas a 'supporter' might only follow a particular team, go to regular matches and be part of the club community. Nowadays you can become a fan of a club while never actually seeing your team play, as my youngest son Tommy will attest – he doesn't like loud noises, which immediately keeps him out of St James' Park on matchdays. In fact, during a recent shopping trip to the Metrocentre, while my husband and our eldest were ensconced in the bosom of the Toon Army, the roar when Newcastle scored could be heard as we emerged into the street. Tommy gave me a knowing look of 'see, loud enough', while also rejoicing at the confirmed goal on my Sky Sports app.

He has been inside St James' Park, however. In fact, he has been in the dressing rooms, the directors' box and has walked down the tunnel, toe-touching the hallowed turf in front of him. Taking part on a stadium tour the day before the final home game of the 2023/24 season was as exciting as it comes for the boys and myself. Mary and Nick were our tour guides, who, with 25 years of working at St James' Park, were the fount of all knowledge. The things they've seen could probably fill a book by itself but it's interesting to note a few here. Like how the away team dressing rooms here are one of the nicest in the leagues – some tactics deployed at other Premier League venues deliberately make the layout an awkward shape or they put a pillar in the middle of it to make it hard for the manager to make eye contact with the whole team at the same time. Others (Nottingham Forest) also put hooks either too high for players to reach (wouldn't it be awful if they had to stretch and pulled a vital muscle) or too low (Southampton) so that they can't sit comfortably without it digging into their backs. The number of showers is also important; unlucky 13 for the away team for some venues, or not enough in others.

The bust of Bobby Robson is far more imposing as you come into the foyer, and plans are underway to increase the size of the away team dressing room, which is currently a bare, grey, tiled room. And there's no clock either. By contrast, the home team dressing room starts filling with players a couple of hours before kick-off, the ghetto blaster that Eddie installed for the players giving each one the opportunity to listen to one or two of their favourite songs as he plays them on a loop so it's not just one person's song choice.

There's a separate training room attached that doubles up as a warming-up zone and a place for Eddie to give one of his many pre-match team talks of the day. Then it's time to walk out, once you've put on your right boots for the match – each player has six depending on what the moisture in the grass is like and therefore what length of stud they use. Moving out into the tunnel, the home team always taking the right side as they head out to the Gallowgate End. It's not a straightforward run-out to the pitch, another psychological ploy that upsets the away team, as they can't see the grass until they're bombarded with the view, the sights, the decibels right at the end of the tunnel, which also signals a point of no return.

There's nothing that describes the noise on matchday at St James' Park. It infiltrates your bones. Doing a stadium tour the day before is both eerily quiet in comparison and a chance to notice all the things that are missed as soon as the starting whistle blows: the flags all being wound around by a team of volunteers and placed on the seats; the pitch, strangely green as the lines haven't been painted on yet; the tables being set in the private boxes; the sign that reminds guests that it's a criminal offence to consume alcohol in view of the pitch.

I have a lot to thank Mary and Nick for in the two hours we spent with them, taking us to areas that will live in the memories of my sons for years to come – playing 'Local Hero' while they walked out through the tunnel, a proud father and sister following behind while I captured the moment forever on video. I also have Mary to thank for the idea of this front cover. My idea of a magpie flying over St James' Park was quickly changed to two magpies when we visited the crest wall. The current club crest is now the oldest in the Premier League (Newcastle have just taken over that accolade from Norwich), a simpler version of the first crest, which had the city's coat of arms emblazoned on the shirts in 1969. But it was when she started talking about the next couple of crests – the 1976 badge, which had the words Newcastle United Football Club in circular form around a solitary magpie and in front of an illustration of the Castle Keep and the River Tyne, and the 1983 club cult classic (which only had a shelf life of five years) and just the letters NUFC with a magpie in the upturned C – that she brought to my attention the problem of one magpie. There's no sorrow with this book and it's also why you have two magpies now flying high on the front cover of this book. Thanks, Mary.

Playing pool in The Strawberry, the landlord said that Eddie Howe had been in a couple of weeks earlier, playing pool and doing some promotion of sorts. A couple of cleaners who work in the stadium were watching and telling their stories of players and history to my son, who came over and told me just as they were leaving about how they'd seen Bruno and how nice Dan Burn is. Everyone we met was a hero to my son, from the punters who told him they hoped he enjoyed the game, to the landlord that asked him his score prediction. And, of course, gave him a vital piece of information: 'Last home game tomorrow, lad, the atmosphere will be electric. Make sure you get there early … five to three!'

The level of exposure of a team nowadays is phenomenal. My sons can watch the chants about Bruno and Gordon from games two years ago from fans who've posted footage online as if they were there. Social media allows players, owners, coaches, backroom staff to upload photos of what they had for breakfast, videos of their children's birthday parties, snapshots of their homes and them at training … the access is endless. It's a level of access that my father-in-law could have only dreamed about when he received his copy of *The Pink* given to him a day after a match – after his big brother had first dibs. Trying to explain that to Henry, what *The Pink* newspaper was, was a trip down memory lane, and one that deserves sharing. *The Pink* reported on all the football matches in the North East, as well as non-league football clubs and grassroots-level news, but it was, of course, Newcastle United that everyone wanted to read about.

'We'd often wait in the pub after a game,' recalled Tony, 'mostly in good spirits after a home win, and then the vendor would come in. He'd probably only make it to the doorway when people would, like, surround him. We'd want to get a copy to see the league table and check scores and, of course, read all about the game we'd just watched.' Having worked in the newspaper industry, I know a thing about deadlines, but to get a report out on a match in a matter of hours after the game was something else. Paul New, the sports editor on *The Chronicle*, also oversaw production on *The Pink* most Saturdays and was well aware of the manic deadlines that ensured fans got their post-match fix:

> At 3pm kick-off time on a Saturday afternoon, you'd have ten blank pages to fill. There would be information coming in from all angles and as the matches progressed, the Newcastle and Sunderland reports would be phoned in to a copy taker. At Thomson House, we could hear the roar of the crowd from St James' Park when a goal was scored – and we knew our Newcastle reporter Alan Oliver would soon be on the line reporting good news. We had to have everything wrapped up and ready to go by 5.05pm, our deadline. The presses were ready to roll downstairs, and the vans and vendors were waiting, but a late goal might mean a major rewrite, and sometimes there might be lengthy injury time, or there might have been a late kick-off. The back page with all the match results and league tables was sent to us complete by the Press Association, and that could be affected by technical problems as the minutes ticked by.

* * *

Neil Armstrong famously once said about a step being simultaneously small and yet gigantic at the same time. The same can be said about a 0-0 draw in a football match. On the surface it doesn't mean a lot, zero in fact. But put a goalless match in the right context and its significance is immeasurable. When Newcastle drew 0-0 with Leicester on 22 May 2023, it was their Armstrong moment. 'Keep it going, keep it going' were the words from Bruno in the changing rooms at half-time. Echoed by similar: 'Same mentality, boys, we've worked so hard this season, boys' from Kieran Trippier. 'Don't be complacent, don't get tired, keep calm' from Dan Burn. While the chants from the crowd were growing in excitement and assurance: 'Tell me ma, ma, ma, I won't be home for tea, we're going to Italy!'

And they were. When the final whistle was blown, Newcastle had secured a Champions League place for the first time in 22 years and the boring result was quickly forgotten in place of the significance of the occasion. Because, of course, the Leicester game, although the point in time that changed the Saudi-owned club's future, was the culmination of hundreds of matches before this cool May evening that helped turn Newcastle's future around.

It was bittersweet that Newcastle's triumph was against a team who'd also faced their moment of glory in the past, one of the greatest sporting stories of all time in fact. Starting the 2015/16 season as 5,000/1 outsiders for the Premier League title, it was probably only diehard, lifelong fans (and one certain gambler, if that's not an oxymoron) who would have ever believed that the Foxes had the capability to win it. In a story that you probably couldn't make up, Leicester (Walkers crisps, Gary Lineker, Engelbert Humperdinck, Red Leicester cheese, that

Leicester!) proved they were a city that was more than just crisps and who were nearly relegated the season before. They managed to lose only three league games all season and pulled off one of the biggest sporting shocks in history. Alan Shearer, speaking at the time, concluded it was the most impressive thing to have ever happened in the game: 'For a team like Leicester to come and take the giants on with their wealth and experience – not only take them on but to beat them – I think it's the biggest thing to happen in football.'

And so it was that Leicester players and fans probably knew what a moment it was for Newcastle. 'We'd had our own moment, we knew what it means to a club that has worked tirelessly in the past, to get to this point,' revealed Foxes fan Lucas.

The Rise of the Magpies might not be the epic short story of such glory, but it's much more than that. And it makes a much greater read. To trace the lineage of success means to focus primarily on the 2022/23 season, pass back to the Mike Ashley era, before volleying over to 2017 and the start of the takeover talks. The 2021/22 season is its own fairy tale because it was unprecedented that a team that had spent the length of time in the relegation zone as the Magpies did would avoid relegation. But with new owners, a new manager, new signings, they did. And now look at them.

Howay the Toon.

Chapter 1

The Ashley Era

'We know if you're not being sincere, we can tell. You can't get much past the fans.'

David

THE ERA of Mike Ashley, although originally full of expectation, full of promise and ultimately and most importantly full of cash, was little in terms of deliverance. Hope can be, as they say, the cruellest emotion of them all, and although the Sports Direct CEO was initially quick to earn the handshakes and the hugs from the fans, buying pints at the local bars and sharing away-day transport with fans, he was the biggest disappointment of them all. The fans know a committed owner when they see one and the resentment started to build over the years. Now if you mention the name Mike Ashley, you're likely to be met with expletives and headshakes.

The reasons for this animosity are numerous and were built on his lack of investment in the team, his disregard for the club's history and traditions and his handling of managerial appointments. He made hasty and ill-informed decisions when it came to hiring and firing managers, resulting in a lack of stability and continuity at the club, with numerous managers coming and going in a short period of time. Ten different managers, to be exact. The constant upheaval and uncertainty hindered the team's progress and made it difficult for any manager to build a successful team and secure success on the pitch. Coupled with Ashley's failure to invest, this meant that there was no spark when it came to signings. His reluctance to splash the cash on quality players to improve the squad was obvious, instead opting for cheap and inexperienced signings. This lack of ambition and investment led to a decline in the performance and reputation of Newcastle United. It was a vicious circle.

Under Ashley's ownership the team often struggled in the lower half of the Premier League table and were relegated twice – in the 2008/09 season and again in 2015/16, although they returned to the top flight both times at the first opportunity by winning the Championship. 'I want to have fun and win some trophies,' said Ashley when he assumed control in 2007. What a joke that statement turned out to be.

I don't want to rehash old ground and, ideally, I know many fans would like to draw a big 'Mike who?' line under that whole period. But I'm reminded again of the new generation of fans now seeing a club with a strong owner, a respected manager and a stability that shouldn't be taken for granted. *The Rise of the Magpies* is all the more poignant when you add the right context of the time their wings were clipped. There's a solidarity among the club and the fans, especially the younger fans who showcase their love of their team, not just by matchday attendance and rundown of the game with their mates afterwards, but by the many channels of social media, chat apps, YouTube channels and gaming platforms that allow this amazing and incomparable fanbase to flourish.

'The name Mike Ashley doesn't mean anything to Henry, it doesn't make his blood run cold and shake his head,' reveals my husband, talking of our 11-year-old supporter son. So, for the purposes of context and a brief history lesson for the younger generation, please indulge me. Mike Ashley bought Newcastle United in May 2007 for a reported £134 million.

> Rob: When he came in, he was like, everything seemed great. He was a millionaire, he had plenty of money and, although no one had heard of him, he came in and bought Newcastle and everything was great. He would go out with fans to nightclubs and buy them drinks and everyone thought it was a breath of fresh air. And he brought back Kevin Keegan, which everyone thought was great!

Geordie hero Kevin Keegan came in as a replacement to Sam Allardyce, a popular move among the fans. Everyone who remembered the 90s remembered when Newcastle United earned the nickname 'the entertainers' for their exhilarating style of play and their ability to captivate fans with their attacking prowess, all under the management of King Kev. That was a time Newcastle became one of the most exciting teams in English football, thrilling spectators with their attacking football and never-say-die attitude, and fans were hoping for a repeat of history.

Cast your minds back to 1992. Keegan, a former England international and, of course, former Newcastle United player, brought a new vision and philosophy to the club. He believed in playing attractive, attacking football that would excite the fans and bring success. Assembling a team of players who'd become the backbone of 'the entertainers', he signed Peter Beardsley, Andy Cole and David Ginola, who'd go on to become fan favourites and play pivotal roles in the team's success. These players were not only skilled footballers but also possessed a flair and creativity and, coupled with an attacking style of play with a high tempo, speed and precision, they were a formidable force.

Probably one of the defining moments of that era came in the 1995/96 season when Newcastle United mounted a title challenge that captured the imagination of football fans across the country. Led by the prolific strike partnership of Alan Shearer and Les Ferdinand, they were the top scorers in the league that season, netting an impressive 66 goals. Despite this impressive haul they missed out on the Premier League title to Manchester United. But the legacy of 'the entertainers' lived on, especially with their never-say-die attitude that resonated with fans, and all this had a lasting impact on the club's identity. Newcastle United became synonymous with attacking football and a never-give-up mentality. The team's spirit and determination became part of the club's DNA. It captivated football fans from around the country, even if they didn't support Newcastle, as my father-in-law recalls.

> Grampy: There was a newfound respect for Newcastle. They became the second-favourite club to lots of people.
>
> You have to remember, this brand of football wasn't known among other clubs and, of course, with matches then starting to be widely televised, people had access to watching Newcastle play this wonderful entertaining style of football.

So it's easy to see why, when Ashley brought back in Keegan in 2007, the fans were buzzing with historical expectation, as John told me:

> We thought with Keegan back, we'd have the best chance of playing exciting football and score lots of goals and be talked about again. We went to St James' to meet Keegan who had Mike Ashley grinning from ear to ear next to him. Ashley could walk on water to all of us then.

But it didn't have the same nostalgic joy that the fans had hoped for. The one-time entertainers of English football were reduced to a grim curiosity. The rest of the country were smug, knowing NUFC's plight was not theirs. Supporters merely endured.

It was very clear very early on that Ashley was running the club exactly how he wanted to, to the detriment of the fans, the players and the team's success.

> Rob: Mike Ashley was only concerned about having Mike Ashley people around him. He brought in Dennis Wise, and let me tell you something, Dennis Wise was hated up here in Newcastle, hated. He was a dirty player, a player who would just wind up the crowd and, out of 50,000 fans at Newcastle, 51,000 hated him.

Former Chelsea midfielder Dennis Wise joined the Magpies in January 2008 as the club's Executive Director of Football, a role that was met with mixed reactions from fans and pundits alike. But Wise laughed in the face of controversy, having had a successful playing career marred by disciplinary issues, so he didn't care in the slightest that his appointment at Newcastle was seen as a bold move by owner Mike Ashley, who believed that Wise's experience and knowledge of the game would help the club.

One of Wise's first tasks was to assist Keegan in the January transfer window. The duo brought in several new players, including the likes of Jonás Gutiérrez and Sébastien Bassong. These signings initially brought a glimmer of hope to the fans but things turned sour as tensions between Keegan and Wise began to rise.

> Rob: Keegan wasn't happy because Dennis Wise tried to get him to sign a player by just watching videos of this player on YouTube! Well, of course, Keegan wouldn't do that, he would send out his own scouts for new players, he would invite them to see them play, he wouldn't just watch videos of someone! When he left, it went downhill from there.

Keegan resigned from his position in September 2008, citing interference from the board as the main reason for his departure. This incident sparked outrage among the fans, who saw Wise as the orchestrator of their beloved Keegan's exit. Wise remained at the club and took on a more prominent role in the footballing side of things, appointing Joe Kinnear as interim manager, a decision that was met with scepticism by many fans and pundits and disappointment by even more fans and pundits alike.

Kinnear's previous managerial experience, which included stints at Wimbledon and Luton Town, didn't inspire confidence in his ability to lead a Premier League club and, from the outset, his time at Newcastle was marred by a series of questionable decisions and public outbursts. In what's now an infamous press conference, he mispronounced the names of several Newcastle players and swore repeatedly (over 65 times to be exact), setting the incompetence tone for his tenure and immediately alienating him from the club's supporters.

Perhaps the most damning aspect of Kinnear's time at Newcastle was the team's relegation from the Premier League in 2008/09. Despite inheriting a squad that had finished 12th the previous season, Kinnear was unable to steer the team clear of the drop zone. Disheartening wasn't the word.

> Isaac: I remember watching week-in, week-out, losing every week. I remember sitting watching us get relegated from the Premier League with my uncle and just being so upset. Even now I just remember how little Mike Ashley did for our club.

Kinnear's transfer dealings during his time at Newcastle were equally underwhelming. While he was given control over player recruitment, he failed to make any significant signings that would improve the squad. Instead, he brought in several mediocre players who failed to make an impact on the team. He was responsible for bringing in the likes of Xisco and Ignacio González, two players who failed to make any significant impact at the club. These signings, along with others, were seen as a waste of money, lacking in ambition and further fuelled the fans' frustration.

Kinnear's management style also came under scrutiny. He was known for his abrasive and confrontational approach, often clashing with players and staff. There was a toxic atmosphere within the club and his inability to build positive relationships with the players and foster a cohesive team spirit was evident in Newcastle's performances, which were consistently uninspiring. It didn't help matters that the likes of Wise and Kinnear, along with Tony Jimenez, a close associate of Ashley who was also involved in the club's operations and played a role in player recruitment, were colloquially known as the 'Cockney Mafia'. The exact composition of this group isn't clear but it's believed that they were all involved in various capacities at Newcastle during Ashley's tenure.

> Rob: They brought in Joe Kinnear, who'd been out of the game. He was in charge of Nottingham Forest, I believe. Why was he in? I have no idea, pet, he was Dennis Wise's friend. Kinnear was manager at Wimbledon when Dennis Wise was a player. Wise was always disliked as a player, and bringing in Joe Kinnear was a joke. He actually tried to sign a player who was on our books but we'd loaned him out, and he couldn't get to grips with some of the players' names. All the Newcastle fans used to call them and Ashley the Cockney Mafia.

The term was often used by Newcastle fans and critics to express their frustration and dissatisfaction with the perceived influence of these individuals over the club. It was a nickname given to the group of London-based businessmen who were believed to have significant influence over the club's operations and decision-making processes. More significantly, these individuals were thought to have no understanding of the club's values and traditions, a sacrosanct value for Geordies. 'Out Cockney Mafia' signs were displayed by fans, particularly during the time Londoner Alan Pardew took over as manager.

Ashley gave him an eight-year contract in 2012, which raised eyebrows, although it confirmed Pardew's status inside Ashley's inner circle. It's important to note that 'Cockney Mafia' is subjective and has been disputed by some individuals associated with the club, but it remains a part of the narrative surrounding Newcastle United during Mike Ashley's ownership.

In April 2009, Wise left Newcastle United by mutual consent, ending a tumultuous period for both the club and the former midfielder. His time at Newcastle will be remembered for the controversies, poor transfer decisions and the strained relationships with managers and fans. But things could only get better, right? This would be a fresh start for everyone and a brighter future for the club, wouldn't it? Not with Ashley still in charge. He was the figurehead for all that was going wrong with the club.

> Alan: I think he was just a ruthless businessman. He put a lot of money into Newcastle but he took a lot out. He ruined the club. He wasn't a football man, he was a businessman and wasn't interested in the football side, the talent or who was playing.

Furthermore, Ashley's lack of transparency and rare communication with the fans was creating a sense of disconnect between the owner and the fanbase, leading to a breakdown in trust and a feeling of being ignored. The fans felt their voices weren't being heard and their concerns, namely that he didn't care about the club, weren't addressed. He appointed golden boy Shearer as interim manager when Kinnear left the club but, with only eight games in charge before the end of the season and no money to buy new players as the transfer window was closed, the club was relegated.

Ashley decided Shearer wasn't cut out to be manager. ('I told him what I thought should happen next,' revealed Shearer, 'and I never heard from him again. All of us were ostracised from the club we used to be. We were alienated. I felt so unwelcome.') Ashley brought in Chris Hughton and renamed Shearer's Bar, the famous drinking place attached to the stadium in honour of the Magpies' leading goalscorer, as Nine Bar.

> Sharon: Ashley made huge profits from the club and all of the fans but none of that money was invested back into Newcastle in the 14-odd years he owned the club. There was no investment in the team, the stadium, the training facilities or coaching. Which ultimately meant no progression for the team in any cup competitions, no hope for the players, who eventually left when fed up of not achieving much, and no hope for the fans.

Sharon's opinion was that he was lining his pockets and the club was just left to survive. Another frustration for Newcastle fans was Ashley's blatant disregard for the club's history and traditions, renaming the stadium from St James' Park to Sportdirect.com@StJames'Park, before rebranding it again to the Sports Direct Arena. This move was seen as a disrespectful and a commercialisation of the club's heritage, showcasing Ashley's selfish agenda, promoting his own business, Sports Direct, over the club's proud and historical identity. The stadium wasn't then, isn't now and never has been just a sporting ground. St James' Park is a symbol of the city's identity and a gathering place for the community. From its humble beginnings as a cricket ground to its transformation into a world-class stadium, St James' Park has witnessed the triumphs and tribulations of the club. It stands as a testament to the city's love for football and remains an iconic landmark in Newcastle upon Tyne.

> Grampy: St James' Park ... it's hard to describe what it is. Whichever direction you go in, it's the first thing you see, it stirs something that's in you. It's iconic because it's well known to everyone, but here's the funny thing, whether you're a home or away supporter, you're proud of it. You're proud of what it represents. And not many clubs can say that about their ground.

The passion and loyalty of fans make St James' Park a bastion, creating an electric atmosphere on matchdays. It's incredible to witness first-hand, and for my son, coming up to watch a game at St James' for the first time, an experience he'll never forget.

> Henry: The songs are loud, Mum, everyone is singing or waving a flag. It felt like I was home, everyone just wanted to be there for the same reason and I was hugging everyone!

Quicker than a hiccup, Henry was part of the Toon Army and submerged in the cauldron of passion, excitement and unwavering support for the home team.

> Isaac: The atmosphere is like music to your ears. As soon as you hear the crowd roar it's like adrenaline

like you have never felt before rush through your body.

It's a sentiment that's echoed far and wide. The passion and energy create an atmosphere that's unmatched in any other club. The chants, flags and sheer volume of noise make the stadium a deafening place for opponents and a serenade for the home team.

The origins of St James' Park can be traced back to the 19th century when a group of cricket enthusiasts formed the Newcastle East End Cricket Club. In 1880, the club decided to add a football section to their organisation, and St James' Park became their home ground. The park was named after a nearby church dedicated to St James and was a modest venue. Six years later Newcastle East End merged with a local club called West End to form Newcastle United. The newly formed club became one of the powerhouses of English football, and St James' Park became their fortress. 'It's the fortress on the hill, it's the first thing you see when you come to Newcastle, our welcome home sign to supporters,' confirms fan Tommy James.

For those who don't know their fortress history (and for those that do, humour us), the Leazes Stand was built in 1905, followed three years later by the Gallowgate End. During the 1920s and 1930s, St James' Park witnessed some of its greatest moments. Under the management of legendary manager Stan Seymour, Newcastle won three league titles and reached the FA Cup Final four times, winning it on three occasions. In 1953, floodlights were installed and a decade later the Milburn Stand was constructed. With a capacity for 52,000, it has not only been a venue for football but has also hosted other sporting events – it's a regular venue for rugby union matches, for example.

Beyond its sporting significance, St James' Park holds a special place in the hearts of the people of Newcastle. The stadium is a symbol of the city's identity and a gathering place for the community, which is why, when Ashley reportedly prioritised his own business interests over the well-being of the club and used the stadium as a platform for advertising his own company, it was a bitter pill for fans to swallow. And how much did he really care about football in the end?

> Rob: Mike Ashley had the money to spend but he didn't buy any players or do anything with his money for the club. He went out and bought Debenhams instead! He's a businessman, I get that, but you don't run a football club and buy Debenhams!

Ashley presided over two of Newcastle's six relegations in their 129-year history, so his departure from the club was met with both relief and optimism by the fans. After a tumultuous tenure as owner marked by a lack of investment, poor decision-making, alienating icons and overpromoting interlopers, spending money begrudgingly and intermittently, and a strained relationship with the fanbase, many supporters saw Ashley's departure as a positive step towards a brighter future for the club. Things can only get better, as the song goes, and they did. They very much did.

Chapter 2

Goodbye Big Mike

'A new era begins …'

NUFC's X (formerly Twitter) account

THE SAUDI takeover of Newcastle United in 2021 was a highly controversial and polarising event that captured the attention of football fans and the media around the world. But we don't need to tell you that.

Yes, it was a monumental moment in the club's history and sent shockwaves throughout the footballing world, but, for supporters, the acquisition of the club by the Saudi Arabian Public Investment Fund (PIF), Amanda Staveley's PCP Capital Partners and the Reuben brothers brought with it nothing but a wave of excitement about the future of the club. 'It was the best thing that could have happened to Newcastle, the very best,' says Irene, a fan. 'It was more than what we could have hoped for.'

This takeover had been a long time coming and several years in the making. The weight of Mike Ashley's reign was weighing heavily on the shoulders of everyone associated with the club and there was an angry impotence among fans. Having been under Ashley's reign and continuously drowning in a sea of despair, talks of a takeover bid were like the lifeboats on the horizon. Underneath all the metaphors, of course, was a strong sense of outrage. So thank goodness for Amanda Staveley, a prominent businesswoman and financier who'd long been associated with hopes for a brighter future for Newcastle United Football Club. Her interest began in 2017 when she led a consortium, which included the PIF, in a bid to take over the club.

However, the Premier League faced a difficult decision in approving or rejecting the Saudi takeover when it was initially brought to them. On one hand, the financial investment promised by the PIF could have significant benefits for Newcastle United and the wider community. The club's infrastructure and facilities could be improved, and there could be a boost to the local economy through increased tourism and investment. But, on the other hand, approving the takeover would send a message that human rights concerns can be overlooked in the pursuit of financial gain. The Premier League had to carefully consider the potential impact on its reputation and values.

The Saudi takeover also brought about concerns regarding the integrity of the sport. The Premier League faced criticism for allowing the acquisition to go through, despite the concerns raised about the new owners. Many argued that the takeover was a clear example of 'sportswashing', a term used to describe the use of sports to divert attention from controversial actions or human rights abuses. This led to calls for greater scrutiny and regulation in the ownership of football clubs.

The Saudi takeover also had wider implications for the Premier League and its relationship with Saudi Arabia. The PIF's involvement in Newcastle United raised questions about the league's commitment to upholding its own values and principles. It also sparked debates about the influence of foreign investment in English football and the potential for a shift in power dynamics within the league.

After months of deliberation and scrutiny, the Premier League ultimately rejected the Saudi takeover of Newcastle United. They cited concerns about the separation of the PIF from the Saudi government and the need for more information on the ownership structure. The decision was met with disappointment by many Newcastle United fans, who'd hoped for a new era of investment and success for their club. It was frustrating, as Newcastle supporters just wanted out from Ashley and were happy to square the circle of being ecstatic about the end of a disastrous era of ownership and the moral implications of a regime like Saudi Arabia controlling their club.

> Grampy: Saudi Arabia weren't the problem at all; the problem was that people thought the Arabs would come in and take over the Premiership. It was going to be the best thing that happened to the club but we were setting a precedent and there was a lack of understanding over the positives and a focus on the negatives.

With the controversial £300 million takeover of Newcastle United axed, Staveley was public in her upset. 'We are heartbroken, obviously,' she said. 'Of course we do [blame the Premier League]. They had a chance, they say we have not answered all the questions and we have done so. But the other clubs in the Premier League didn't want it to happen.'

This dig was in reference to a certain London club. One club that had been particularly vocal about the issue was Tottenham Hotspur, who'd expressed their concerns and opposition to the proposed deal. Their reasons, on the surface, were seemingly admirable and many thought they were voicing the views of clubs in general, or were rooted in concerns about human rights, financial imbalance and potential political influence. Tottenham believed that the values and principles of the Premier League should be upheld and that allowing a regime with a poor human rights record to own a club would be detrimental to the league and the sport.

The Saudi regime has often been criticised for its poor human rights record, including issues such as the treatment of women, freedom of speech and the persecution of political dissidents. Tottenham not only believed that allowing a club to be owned by a regime with such a record would go against the values and principles of the Premier League, but were also concerned about the potential financial power that the Saudi consortium would bring to Newcastle United. The PIF that was leading the takeover bid had significant financial resources at its disposal, which could have led to Newcastle potentially becoming a dominant force in terms of financial resources. This could ultimately have a detrimental effect on the competitiveness of the league, as well as the ability of other clubs to compete on a level playing field.

Another issue that Tottenham raised was the potential influence that the Saudi government could have on the running of the club. There were concerns that the Saudi regime could use the club as a tool for political influence and propaganda. This could have wider implications for the integrity of the league and the sport as a whole.

But many thought that Tottenham's opposition to the Saudi takeover of Newcastle United was based more on self-interest and rejection.

> Grampy: Tottenham were against the takeover because the Saudis hadn't approached them. Tottenham wanted to be bought but they'd been refused.

He was right. Spurs nearly sold to the Saudis back in 2019 but they'd been rejected, and a supposed billion-pound takeover hadn't gone through.

But for Tynesiders the dream of supporting one of England's richest clubs did go through, and on 8 October 2021 Mike Ashley completed the sale of the club to a consortium backed in part by the PIF. 'It was like when Abu Dhabi consortium bought Man City or when Qatar bought PSG [Paris Saint-Germain],' recalled Doug. 'Newcastle now had bloody wealthy owners!'

The Saudi takeover was met with excitement and optimism by many Newcastle United fans. The potential injection of significant financial resources from the PIF promised a new era of investment and ambition for the club. Supporters hoped that this influx of funds would enable the team to compete with the top clubs in the Premier League and challenge for major honours. The prospect of a wealthy and ambitious owner was seen as a welcome change from the previous regime of Mike Ashley, whose lack of investment and ambition had frustrated fans for years. Far too many years.

> Rob: The takeover? I was buzzing, absolutely buzzing. I was so happy. We just wanted the team to have the chance to try again. I've been to matches on and off for 50 years. I haven't seen them win anything at all. When the consortium took over the club, we were suddenly the team that tries, we didn't want to be relegated anymore.

But it was the new owners' hope to restore the club's reputation and standing in the footballing world that brought a sense of pride back to the community.

> Sharon: The new owners have the right perspective and drive to improve the club and the facilities for all and make a profit. I think within weeks of taking over, improvements in every area of what's Newcastle United were announced. Better communication with all is a great start. I think something like £38 million was quoted to be needed just to bring the club up in line with other big clubs in the Premier League, but just sprucing up the ground and updating things around the stadium gives the fans a lift. It was a fresh new start!

When the new owners took over, Newcastle were sitting 19th in the Premier League in 2021/22. First and foremost, the PIF, with an estimated worth of over £320 billion, promised to invest heavily in the team with the aim of transforming it into a powerhouse, both on and off the pitch.

On the sporting front, the takeover meant ambitious plans for Newcastle United, with the new owners expressing their desire to turn the club into a global brand, capable of challenging for major honours both domestically and in European competitions. They promised to invest in world-class players, top-tier coaching staff and state-of-the-art training facilities. This raised expectations among fans, who'd endured years of mediocrity and underachievement under the previous ownership.

Some fans were uncertain.

> Alan: I was dubious of the new owners when they came in. I still am, to be honest. They have more money than any other Premier League club put together but you can't spend it.

Whereas for others, the owners signified a winning mentality.

> Rob: I've been to Wembley three times. I've been to finals and I've never seen them win anything. So when the Saudis came in, they don't play second best, they play to win, they want the best.

One of Staveley's main hopes for Newcastle United was to bring success to the club with the ability to attract top-quality players and managers. But success along with stability – that all-important element that had been missing for the past 14 years. Newcastle United's fans have been patient a long time and Staveley and the new owners knew they had to satisfy supporters' expectations on a grand scale. 'We just wanted to win games for the past 14 years, we just wanted an owner who showed support and wanted to give their all to this one-club city to show its potential,' confirmed Rory. 'But now … Well, now the sky's the limit! I remember hearing talks that Mbappé would be coming over the Tyne Bridge in those early days!'

Newcastle was a feverish place in the hours after the confirmation, and Staveley said, 'Of course we have the same ambitions as Manchester City and PSG in terms of trophies, absolutely, but that will take time.'

They had time to prepare for who they wanted in the transfer window, which was a couple of months away, but the most pressing item on the agenda was who was going to take the lead from the front; who was going to take charge of the team?

We all know how this ends. Even Steve Bruce knew. He was unpopular with supporters, hadn't won a league game all season and spoke like a man bracing himself for dismissal as soon as the takeover was announced. Plus, any new regime always wants their own man for the job, and the consortium knew they had to choose wisely. But who?

The names doing the rounds at the time were vast and fanciful because there was no limit to the imagination of fans and pundits. Initial names doing the rounds ranged from Leicester City's Brendan Rodgers, AS Roma's Jose Mourinho, to Rangers' Steven Gerrard, and the still loved Rafa Benítez, who was now at Everton. Other names being whispered about were Antonio Conte, a coach who won the Premier League with Chelsea but was known for being quite high maintenance, Frank Lampard, Roberto Martinez and Eddie Howe. 'We didn't know who they were going to pick, we just knew that Bruce had to go,' confirmed Matt.

Dismissing Bruce was easy. But who next? That was the million-pound question …

Chapter 3

Eddie's Boys

'Eddie Howe doesn't get angry like the other football managers I see on TV, like Arteta – Arsenal's manager – he's always calm and kind, even when Newcastle lose or do something wrong. He always talks about the positives, not the negatives for Newcastle.'

Tommy Smith, aged nine

ON 8 November 2021, Eddie Howe was confirmed as head coach of Newcastle United, just one month after the takeover was formally announced. His appointment was seen as a statement of intent from the club's new ownership group and injected a renewed sense of hope and optimism into the club. It sent a clear message to the fans, the players and the wider footballing world that Newcastle United were ready to compete at the highest level, they had ambition and wanted success, and Howe was the right man for the job. There was still a school of thought that appointing a footballing fundamentalist like Howe for a huge club in the thick of a relegation battle wasn't a good choice. But then they probably hadn't met the man.

Born on 29 November 1977, in Amersham, Eddie Howe began his football journey as a player with a professional career at Bournemouth as a central defender. His playing career was cut short due to a knee injury, but little did he know that this setback would lead him to a new calling as a manager.

Appointing Eddie ended a hectic 33 days of turmoil for Newcastle and the new owners. Five days after the takeover was completed, Amnesty International wrote to Premier League CEO Richard Masters requesting an 'urgent' meeting on proposed changes to football's takeover rules, following Newcastle's change of ownership. Then on 17 October the first game of the new era of Newcastle's ownership kicked off, and 90 minutes later their players left the pitch having been defeated 3-2. It was Steve Bruce's 1,000th game in management but the pressure was now on. Three days later, on 20 October, Bruce left the club by mutual consent. The club's official statement read:

> After being informed of the news in person by Amanda Staveley and Mehrdad Ghodoussi, the players continued to prepare for Saturday's Premier League trip to Crystal Palace under the guidance of Graeme Jones – who will lead the team on an interim basis – and fellow coaches Steve Agnew, Stephen Clemence, Ben Dawson and Simon Smith.

Bruce's departure was met with jubilation from the fans, who'd grown increasingly frustrated with his tenure as manager. His time at the club was marked by a lack of success on the pitch and a style of play that failed to excite the supporters. In short, he wasn't liked, wasn't respected and wasn't giving fans what they wanted.

'He kept us in the bottom half of the Premier League,' confirmed Ethan. 'He never wanted the players to attack, he never showed any ambition and he always seemed to be keeping us stale at the bottom of the table.'

The final straw for many fans came early in 2021, in the form of a humiliating defeat to Sheffield United, who were bottom of the league at the time. While Sheffield United fans celebrated their first win of that season, Toon Army fans were hanging their heads under the weight of no win in their last six games. This lack of fight and passion displayed by the team was seen as a reflection of Bruce's leadership, and when he left – mutual consent, nudge, nudge, wink, wink – the hope of a new manager with a vibrant personality and the ambition and drive to bring a style of attacking football and mentality that the club is renowned for was all they wanted. Was that too much to ask?

On 21 October, a day after Bruce's departure, the new owners met with Paulo Fonseca, one of the candidates touted as his replacement, who'd taken an early lead as the bookies' favourite. Linked with Tottenham Hotspur over the course of the summer, Fonseca was currently without a club after leaving AS Roma in June following two years in charge of the Italians. Newcastle liked the look of him; on paper he was everything that was needed to bring a bit of excitement to St James' Park and, despite his relatively young age, he'd bring with him a wealth of experience and an impressive win rate of over 50 per cent from his time in the Italian capital. And he represented an entertaining brand of football.

But nothing was announced, and two days later Newcastle missed out on another win with an away draw against Crystal Palace. A Callum Wilson equaliser meant they didn't have to leave with their heads hung too low, picking up one point and stopping the losing streak, but they were still sitting in 19th position, three points from safety. The match also drew lots of unwanted attention due to the home fans being very vocal and visual in their attack on Newcastle's new owners. A complaint was made and the Met Police issued a statement:

> On Saturday 23 October, a member of the public contacted the police to raise concerns about a banner displayed at the Crystal Palace vs Newcastle match at Selhurst Park. Following an assessment, officers have concluded that no offences have been committed. No further action will be taken.

The banner was graphic and showed a man wearing traditional Arab clothing with the letters PIF on his robe, wielding a blood-stained sword. But its protest was legitimate according to Ronan Evain, the executive director of Football Supporters Europe. In an interview with *The Guardian* he said it was legitimate for football fans from other teams to raise questions about the takeover:

> It was a perfectly acceptable form of protest, it was based on facts. I don't think the accusation of racism made any sense in that regard. It's legitimate that fans of other clubs raise criticism of this takeover. It is another superpower in the world of football which will ruin the competitive balance of the league. If you're a fan of a team in the same league at some point in the year you're going to be attending a game against a team owned by one of the world's worst human rights offenders. If that's a topic you care

> about, it's only legitimate you exert your freedom of expression within the boundaries of the law.

On 29 October, there was still no news on a manager but still lots of headlines about the takeover and the new owners. The Premier League agreed to meet with Amnesty International, who were pressing them to agree that the owners' and directors' test includes rules on human rights violations. A day later, Newcastle's dreams of a new era slipped a little out of grasp when they lost 3-0 to Chelsea. Their interim manager Graeme Jones, who'd worked with the team when Bruce was in charge, had put together a five-day training programme for players ahead of the clash but his tactics weren't enough. Jones was liked by the players, especially Callum Wilson, who had, the previous season, openly praised his tactical awareness:

> I think Graeme Jones coming in as a coach [in January] definitely complemented the manager because he's a little bit more tactically aware and up to date, whereas the manager has his different strengths and attributes. When you see the results towards the back end of the season and the way we were in games, we had more of a style and philosophy. That will happen from the start of the season with a good coach around to help out the previous coaches.

Being a caretaker manager is no easy ride, but Jones was well liked and his philosophies respected. 'As long as you're fair with your players and always honest – no matter how blunt or brutal – they'll accept it. Then once they accept it, they start to flourish,' Jones revealed in an article for *Coaches Voice* in 2019.

> Grampy: Jones was taken on by Ashley to assist Steve Bruce, and Jones immediately started improving training and tactics in the team. It soon became apparent that Bruce didn't like the popularity that Jones was gaining within the team and fanbase. Jones wasn't often pitch-side, but watching the games from the stands.

In the *Coaches Voice* article, Jones also talked about his playing career, including the impact on his mental health when he was released by Millwall at the age of 18:

> I found work as an insulation engineer. Putting insulation on pipes while grafting in non-league football. That grounding taught me the power of being real. It allowed me to evaluate myself and what I wanted in life. What I wanted was to coach.

The plumbing and heating world's loss was football management's gain, and Jones took a community coaching role at Newcastle United, describing how he'd 'put cones out and coached kids in Tyneside's suburbs', which gave him the coaching bug and convinced him that he had something to offer. Then, when he began to coach the under-14s for Middlesbrough, he said, 'Every session, I went in with the confidence that I could understand and improve the players I was working with. It's a belief that I've never lost.'

> Rob: Graeme Jones did a better job at Newcastle than Bruce, I think. I also think that's how he got the job in Gareth Southgate's England coaching staff, as he was brilliant for Newcastle.

While the new owners had wiped the slate clean with Bruce's departure, Newcastle were still adrift in the relegation zone. Everyone knew that the next permanent managerial appointment would arguably be the most important since the arrival of Kevin Keegan in February 1992 when they were staring into the abyss of the Third Division. Fans were sharing their thoughts on who they wanted to take over the role, with the likes of Eddie Howe and Antonio Conte joining the bookies' favourite Paulo Fonseca, plus the likes of Wayne Rooney, Frank Lampard and Graham Potter.

On 3 November, Villarreal manager Unai Emery publicly confirmed that Newcastle were interested in hiring him but he rejected the offer. There had been a flurry of stories in the past few days over Emery, a former ex-Arsenal head coach, taking over the Toon reins; however, the Spaniard, on a post on social media, distanced himself from the role and made a statement saying he was '100 per cent committed' to his job at Villarreal: 'I am grateful for the interest of a great club, but even more grateful to be here.'

Coincidentally, three years later, when his commitment to Villarreal had deserted him and his allegiance with Aston Villa began, he made a point of not shaking the hand of assistant Toon boss Jason Tindall after Newcastle beat his team 3-1. 'If someone doesn't want to shake my hand at the end of the game, then I'm not in control of that,' said Tindall. 'I wouldn't personally do that myself, whereas some people act differently when they win compared to when they lose.' Maybe it was just a little sour grapes with Emery that he hadn't taken the job?

Howe had been up against the man in the final stages of interview and knew Emery was the clear favourite for the owners. He told Alan Shearer in an interview, laughing about that situation:

> I found out it was a no and they were going for Unai. When I found out it was down to us both, I could understand the club's decision, because you've got someone who's worked in the top leagues in Europe for a long period of time, so it was almost like I had no chance of winning that fight. But the rest is history.

That it is, Eddie, that it is!

And what about Paulo Fonseca? It had gone quiet on the once favourite, although, according to Spanish football pundit Guillem Balague, Fonseca also believed he was a favourite of the new owners too. Balague told BBC Radio 5 Live in 2021:

> Paulo Fonseca had three interviews with the decision-makers at Newcastle. It got to a point where he thought he was going to be the chosen one. When they realised, or thought or assumed that Unai Emery was going to be the one, they went back to Paulo Fonseca and said, 'No, sorry, it's not going to be you.' He was that close, or at least he thought he was that close to getting it.

So what now? Or rather, who now? Well, glad you asked. On 4 November, Eddie Howe became the front-runner for the position. Very quickly the former Bournemouth coach was heavily discussed on the fans' forum.

Howe's path into management wasn't predicted, most notably by the man himself, who said in an interview in 2021,

'I was sort of thrust into management at Bournemouth, I didn't seek it. But I took the challenge and gave it my all.' After retiring as a player, Howe took up coaching and, in 2008, at the age of 31, he was appointed as the manager of AFC Bournemouth, a club that was struggling in the lower divisions.

Under Howe's guidance, Bournemouth experienced a remarkable rise through the ranks, achieving promotion to the Premier League in 2015. He stayed with them until August 2020 when they were relegated, then took a year out. It was by mutual consent, and Howe, who'd kept the Cherries in the Premier League for five seasons, knew it was time to go:

> In management, you do not have an infinite amount of time in one job. There is a time where people have probably had enough of you, to be honest. I am talking about the players. So, you have to do one of two things, either consistently change the players, or the manager has to leave. I always think there's a shelf life for a manager and I'd probably reached that point where, for the football club, I needed to move on really. I never felt I'd lost control. I was incredibly frustrated that season. I felt we had a good squad of players. But anything that could go wrong did go wrong, and we had crippling injuries. If you look at some of the teams I had to put out, we were constantly playing catch-up.

The fact that Howe penned an address to the supporters on his departure speaks volumes about the level of respect and gratitude he had for the Cherries fans and how much they meant to him. In a 1,209-word open letter, Howe said:

> I now join you as a Bournemouth supporter and will be willing the club on in what I am sure will be a successful future. Bournemouth will always be in my heart, but I firmly believe that now is the right time for the club to have a change. I have always ensured that every decision I have ever made as manager has been in the best interests of the club and its supporters, and this is no different. I'll now be taking some time away during the summer break to enjoy some quality time with my family and I am looking forward to the next chapter in my life.

It had been 16 months since he'd last taken a seat in a dugout but Howe admitted in his first press conference at Newcastle that a long period out of the game was always going to be the plan:

> I said I was going to take a year out. It didn't matter what job came up in that year. I felt I needed to reset and recharge. I wanted to educate myself and take myself away from the thought of taking a job and commit to my family for a period of time, and then commit to coming back better. Even in work, that's always been my focus, self-improvement. I was doing that on a day-to-day basis while in work but I think it's much clearer when you're out of work and you're out of the emotions that football management can bring.
>
> You can take yourself away into a different place mentally. I've been out and about here there and everywhere and I think I sit here now a better manager than I was, even though people would say I've been out of the game and question that, but, for

> me, I'm more relevant and more in touch than I've ever been in terms of what's going on at the top level.

Was being out of a football for so long a concern for fans? For some, including my husband, Chris, it didn't fill him with a great confidence, as he told me one evening over dinner.

> Chris: I wasn't too sure about him at first because I didn't really know who he was. The only thing was that he'd been out of the game for a whole year. And I'm sure the last time he did anything, his team got demoted. I wasn't that confident with him. I was expecting someone a lot bigger to come in, a bigger name because they had the money. But they chose Eddie, and my lack of knowledge was that they were trying to stay up and Eddie was the man to keep them up and he did just that. So I couldn't ask for more.

It was a similar story for others; the unknown was the worry.

> Callum: I'd not heard of him, I was hoping for Mourinho. I had to ask my dad about him, and when he told me he'd been with Bournemouth and did great things there and that he'll know what to do with us too, I felt happier.

But what perhaps my husband and others didn't know at the time was that Howe was using every spare moment – after taking time with his family – to work on himself. To work on his knowledge. 'I had all my diaries, feet tall if you piled them up,' he later revealed. 'Someone would say,

"Give me a training session," and I'd reply, "Give me about 20 minutes and I'll find you one!'"

In an interview with Alan Shearer, Howe revealed that as well as feeding himself with knowledge of the game in his 15-month break, he too felt that he needed to find the right club for him, not just jump at any offer that came his way:

> I didn't know what the right club looked like, it was strange. I needed to be really believe in the project I was going to take on. And having left a club that was very, very special to me, it suddenly hit me – I don't actually know what I'm looking for in my next challenge. I turned down a lot of jobs for that reason. Unless Newcastle had come along, which was immediately the one, I don't know where that would have happened. Celtic was the one job I'd been offered that really appealed but the issue was my staff. I felt that if I was to come into a pressured job like that, I needed to go in with a sense of stability. I needed my staff with me and we couldn't get them together.

In November 2021, his name having been touted around for the past month, Eddie Howe was officially appointed the manager of Newcastle, and co-owner Amanda Staveley said they'd been 'incredibly impressed' by Howe throughout what had been a 'rigorous recruitment process'. Eddie Howe recalls of the interview process:

> You never quite know how you're perceived. I'm presenting not so much on the team but on my method of work and 'this is what I'll do'. One of my

> biggest passions is player development and trying to hone in on making them the best they can be. And then you're waiting for a bit of feedback, you're thinking how did that go?!

Describing him as a 'passionate' and 'dynamic' coach and 'a great fit for what we are trying to build here', Eddie's first game in charge was set to be a home fixture against Brentford on 20 November. Having watched the 1-1 draw against Brighton from the stands, Eddie was aware of the level of responsibility he was facing. 'This is a wonderful opportunity, but there is also a lot of work ahead of us,' he told Newcastle United's official website, referring to his inheriting a team sitting 19th in the table, five points from safety after 11 games:

> I am eager to get on to the training ground to start working with the players. I would like to thank the club's owners for this opportunity and thank the club's supporters for the incredible welcome they have already given me. I am very excited to begin our journey together. It is an incredible moment in my life. The pull of the club is huge. The size of the club, the history of the club. Yes, I've had lots of other options, but I wanted to take my time and really utilise my time away from the game. I feel refreshed, energised and ready to start work. I'll give everything to the job. I'll commit 100 per cent every single day to try and bring success to Newcastle for everybody connected with the club.

Howe was quick to lay out his immediate plans for the squad, having had a similar experience on the south coast:

> My experiences of Bournemouth were so unique. From the first season that I had trying to keep the club in the football league and the existence of the club being under threat, that's huge pressure. I really felt that pressure and I lived it every day. What a great education as part of your first job and taking those expectations on your shoulders. I've learned so much from that. The transfer market isn't the only solution to success. Those principles have lasted with me to this point now and I think that will help me so much in this job.

As his press conference was completed at St James' Park, Howe was mobbed by a crowd of Newcastle fans who were chanting his name and asking for pictures.

He confirmed:

> It's been absolutely incredible. The level of excitement, the level of respect shown to me and the level of interest in the team and the players and the club, it's a new experience for me. It's something that I will relish and will really buy into that culture that is here, how everyone thinks of their football club, and I will try and treat the football club as if the club was my own and do the best for the team and the supporters.

Interestingly, Howe, when returning to Bournemouth in 2023 when Newcastle faced the Cherries, was unable to gauge how he'd feel stepping out into the Vitality Stadium. 'The emotional side is difficult to predict how I'll feel walking out into a stadium I know so well and so many people I know so well,' he said in a press conference before the game. Again, such a few words cementing what we know about a man who shows nothing but respect at every opportunity.

It wasn't just Bournemouth's rise to thc top flight that endeared Howe to the Newcastle faithful, it was his attitude to training that people liked. Former Newcastle striker Alan Shearer was a fan, and said in an interview on BBC Radio 5 Live:

> They have a guy who knows the league, who knows what it's like in that position. He understands the league and what a big club Newcastle are and he'll come back energised. It's a very wise signing.

Howe was known for his humility, his work ethic and his unwavering commitment to his players and the club, and as a manager who leads by example, always willing to put in the hard work and go the extra mile for his team. He was seen as a solid, relentless and detailed man and, although an outsider, was also seen as Newcastle's saviour. Forming a strong bond with and among his squad was another of the hallmarks of Howe's time at Bournemouth, particularly on the journey to the Premier League. Bournemouth became united by a common goal under Howe, part of which was playing for their fans. Newcastle is a club that requires a manager to tap into the passion of the supporters and forge a strong bond between them and the team

'He spends a lot of time getting to know his players, and the great thing he did at Bournemouth was he really tapped into the history of the club,' said former Cherries player Tommy Elphick. 'He made us proud to wear the shirt, and got us playing in a way that resonated with the fans.'

That latter part – the playing style – is also key to getting fans onside. Bournemouth stayed in the Premier League not by playing reactive, counter-attacking football, but by getting on the front foot, and Eddie had similar plans for Newcastle. This was a big contribution to the excitement surrounding Howe's appointment – his commitment to playing attractive and attacking football was something that those in Tyneside craved. Throughout his managerial career, Howe has emphasised the importance of playing an attacking brand of football, with an emphasis on possession, creativity, flair, ambition and high-intensity pressing.

In his first interview after being appointed head coach, he said, 'I love to attack, be on the front foot, play with speed. I want to see fast and dynamic players, playing as a team, not individuals. We want to impose ourselves on the opposition, not wait for the opposition to impose themselves on us.'

> Rob: Eddie Howe was definitely well liked but nobody expected him for us, that was the thing. No one was expecting Eddie to come in, they were expecting big Mourinho and then Eddie comes in. But although he was a surprise addition when he did come in, he went in and spoke to all the players individually. I knew him from Bournemouth and I thought he was a good English manager when he came. I didn't know much else about him, but he's come in and, what he did, he went and met all the players individually, with their wives and their kids, and sat and talked to them as a person, not a player, as a person. He spent time and chatted to their families, getting to know their interests, the kids' birthdays, he wanted to know everything about the players and that's why he has the togetherness with the players, because he has respect and he cares.

Having met former Bournemouth captain Simon Francis on a previous book idea, I was keen to know more about Eddie firsthand and what experiences Simon had with his former boss. Thank you to him for sharing some personal and professional anecdotes on Howe, which I think you'll agree help confirm what we know about the man and his ability to affect any player he works with:

> I had an amazing relationship with Eddie. The first day he joined the football club, the first thing you normally expect from a new manager is a meeting to explain the philosophy that they want to bring to the club. First thing Eddie did was say, 'Let's go down to the beach.' We went down to the beach and took an hour's walk, and he went round to every single player individually and he'd clearly done his homework as new managers should do on the squad that they take over, and every player he had four or five minutes with and spoke about what he really likes, what he expects and the standards he wants to set.
>
> And then he came to me, and from struggling in League One, which we were at the time, and me not having a lot of confidence, he instilled a belief in me on that very first day. He said to me, 'You're going to be my starting right-back, I believe you're going to be the best in the league and I'm going to get you to that level. You've got to trust me, you've got to believe in that yourself and we can do it together.' And from that first day, I thought, *Yep, this is the right man for this job, this squad we have, he's going to be brilliant.*
>
> The training session after that was 100 miles an hour, the quality was brilliant, you could tell the lads just wanted to try and impress him as they knew he

was a special manager. And that was just the first day, and something I'll never forget.

Every time one of the players had a baby, he'd call them into his office. I had Jude, my little boy, at the time when he was manager. I already had Hallie, so when Jude came along, and he's got three boys of his own, he sat me down and we talked about family for half an hour, nothing about football. He asked me how much family meant to me and how much it impacts my football career and he gave me a book that he'd bought when he had his eldest child, and the book he'd read his eldest boy every night at bedtime. And it was about a father and son, a football-related story, and that was an emotional one, but that felt special, with every player who had a baby, calling them into the office. Giving them a book and speaking about family for half an hour, not football, was just a sign of the man that he was.

As a man manager, being able to manage a group of individuals, which he did regularly, definitely the best manager I've worked with, and from purely a manager and players relationship perspective, that comes from his ability to be able to coach individuals every single day on the training ground. He was first in every day, obviously, being manager, and he was always the last off the training ground too. So often you'll see now, training is done and managers go in and you see players do extra bits on their own. Eddie would wait out there until every single player had individual improvement bits from the session. So he'd go round and say, 'Anyone want to do any extra work?' Literally put himself round to work with individuals, which means you could never say, oh, the manager

> doesn't want to improve, doesn't want to work. And that was the only reason he did it. He did it because he genuinely had a passion for improving players, and you can see the impact he's had at Newcastle when he went in there and the improvement straightaway with players, who previously at Newcastle hadn't been standing out or performing to their potential.
>
> But as we know, he's a coach who does that unbelievably and maximises every single player's potential. Which you can see happened at Bournemouth, League One players who didn't believe, didn't have the confidence or didn't think they had the ability to play Premier League football, and then Eddie came in and focused on getting them in the right mindset to improve. Eddie was the right kind of coach that wanted you to improve and you wanted to improve every single day you worked with him. And every training session was a chance to learn. There was never a session where I thought, *That was easy, I could have done that at 20 per cent.* He always asked questions of you every single day, so he always made sure that everyone was engaged and alert to what we were trying to improve.

In addition to his managerial abilities, Howe's reputation as a man of integrity and professionalism has also endeared him to the Newcastle United faithful. Throughout his career, as revealed by Simon, he has been praised for his work ethic, attention to detail and dedication to his craft. He's known for his humility and his ability to build strong relationships with his players, fostering a positive and cohesive team spirit. These qualities make him a perfect fit for a club that values hard work, loyalty and a strong team ethos, as Howe himself explained in an early interview at his new club:

> I want to create an environment where people want to come in and work, a team spirit, a sense that we're in it together. I want the players to bond, to work with them and not against them. I'm hands-on, and it's all about care. Showing you care about people. Going that extra mile and show them that all we can be is just be us.

It wasn't just Howe's tactical acumen that would have the potential to win over the Toon Army. Here was an English manager who was respected and liked, and the Newcastle faithful were ready to welcome him home.

> Isaac: I think Eddie has been perfect as a manager for Newcastle; because of our new takeover we needed someone to gel the team together.

Interestingly, Howe confessed in an interview that, takeover or not, he'd have still taken the job, had it been on offer:

> I wanted to take on a challenge. It was never one I could turn down. Even though you look at the table and we knew it was going to be very, very difficult. But it was all about the size of the club, the history, the optimism of the supporters in that sense of wanting a style of play, wanting to be entertained. I felt I could try and deliver that. The takeover was a bonus for me, in that there was going to be backing, but it wasn't the reason I took the job. I would have taken the job anyway because of the fans and the

> history and the chance to leave a positive mark at a club that has this incredible stature in the game. I wanted to do something to affect people in a city which has that image of 'the entertainers' and to try and recapture that.

Howe's connection to the local community has further endeared him. Under his leadership, Bournemouth played an attractive and attacking style of football, earning them plaudits and a reputation as a team that punched above their weight, and his ability to develop young players and get the best out of his squad was evident. It's been the same here. He understands the importance of the club to the city and its people, and he embraces the responsibility that comes with being the manager – being actively involved in community initiatives and showing a genuine desire to give back to the fans who support the club week-in, week-out.

They appreciate Howe's ability to develop young talent. Throughout his managerial career he has shown a knack for nurturing and improving young players, giving them opportunities to shine on the big stage. This aligns perfectly with the values of the Newcastle United academy, which has a rich history of producing talented players. Howe revealed to Alan Shearer:

> I love the fact it's all about Newcastle. I love that intensity. When I say I want to unite the club, I really mean it. Celebrating our past, celebrating past players, managers, heroes of the club, that has to be part of what you do. You want players to look at it and go, 'I want to be the next Alan Shearer, I want to be talked about.'

My son revealed his thoughts on Howe one bedtime.

> Henry: Newcastle are lucky to have him. I love him. He's so calm, he doesn't seem to get nervous very often and he's very kind. I like that. I watch a lot of his press conferences and he's always very calm. He's never angry and I like that.

It's a sentiment agreed by the army of the Toon and my father-in-law.

> Grampy: Eddie Howe has earned being our manager. When he was first mentioned there were plenty of other managers in the hat too and personally I didn't want Howe to take over Newcastle. I wanted a flamboyant manager, nothing personal against him, like. But within a month of taking over, my mind was changed by him and his attitude.

Full disclaimer, Grampy never likes to admit he's wrong.

It's going to be fairly easy to conclude this chapter by saying that Howe is a manager who embodies the values and aspirations of the club, and he's a beloved figure among the Toon Army. From his playing days to his managerial career, Howe has captured the hearts of Newcastle fans with his positive style of play, his engaging character and his connection to the local community. Everyone is hopeful that his appointment will mark the beginning of a successful and exciting chapter in the club's history. On paper it seems it will: Howe is a hands-on coach with a reputation for playing attacking football but also someone who cares deeply for his players and is capable of rallying a strong squad. Sounds perfectly alreet to us, pet.

Chapter 4

Getting the Flock Together

'Great leaders don't set out to be a leader … they set out to make a difference. It's never about the role – always about the goal.'

Anon

'WHEN YOU think about the mess he inherited from Bruce and Ashley …' sighs my husband, deep in thought, 'Eddie couldn't afford to sit around and not push the team, he needed to come out all guns blazing.'

Evoking an image of a chaps-wearing Howe riding over the Tyne Bridge with his trusty brigade of players behind him ready to stand off against all opposition is an impressive plot for any heroic tale. But in a twist you just couldn't make up, a national pandemic that was still lingering was going to put paid to Howe's debut. Having tested positive for coronavirus the day before Newcastle took on Brentford at St James' Park, Howe had to watch from the comfort of his hotel room. But even though he wasn't there on the sidelines, they say a leader is someone that knows the way, goes the way and shows the way, and

Eddie had, in the past two weeks, been the guy on the ground with his players, showing them there was another way to what they'd been experiencing. That there was a way to escape the bottom of the table. That there was time to turn things around.

The most important thing to consider now was that Howe knew that connection was crucial – creating an energy for his players to feel seen, heard and valued was going to be key to getting this Newcastle side back on track. So when it came to their first match, it didn't matter that he wasn't on the sidelines with them because he was in their heads, their minds and their hearts when they stepped out on to the pitch. Okay, wow, even I get a little caught up in the emotion of it all. Let's head back to when Howe first joined, and the two weeks he had to bring the team together and get training.

His first day, and every one thereafter, was spent drilling home the message 'we train as we play'. That's what the soundtrack from the training pitches was describing. Others said it was like 'pre-season', in that players were returning home from their sessions ready for their bed, as the gaffer had made changes to the training that would extract an extra 'two or three per cent' from the players. 'We are not jogging!' he screamed on that first day. That was an understatement. There were beep tests, there were short, sharp exercises, but nothing boring or repetitive. 'Intense' was a word that kept coming from behind the training gates. 'If you think you're maxed out, you're not' was a popular saying of his.

But Eddie had done his homework. When he left Bournemouth he'd put together a 500-page programme of his training sessions, so he hit the ground running with the players, setting new expectations and standards of punctuality, dress code and eating together. He took all the team to a restaurant for a staff-bonding evening but alcohol was strictly off-limits. There was no rest. It was reported that Eddie's working day started at 7am and would finish around 7pm. He laughed that he hadn't seen Newcastle 'in daylight yet'.

He had lots of plans and he wanted to make lots of changes. One of them that went down particularly well was moving a training stint to St James' Park so that the team could visualise their encounter with Brentford. It was a clever tactic. If you're going to get your players to apply themselves, you need to do it in the exact parameters in which you hope to fit. It was a good move. And even though Eddie himself didn't ever slate the idea that he'd inherited a group of … er … players not quite at their peak of physical fitness, there were one or two in the camp that were happy to make comparisons between their old and new regime.

Callum Wilson, now at Newcastle, had been signed by Howe for just £3m from Coventry City when in charge at Bournemouth. Wilson said in an interview with *The Chronicle* that he remained indebted to Howe, and how Newcastle fans had the right to be excited when he joined the Tyneside club:

> When somebody has helped you so much in your career and gave you the platform in the past to go out and showcase your talent and perform, you're grateful. We have such a good relationship anyway, but our paths have crossed again. Having worked with him in the past, when you're working together, you go on a journey. You get initial success, and then it's a positive spiral effect and that leads on to

> everybody buying into that style of play, buying into the work ethic and buying into the culture. Then it breeds more success and that's what the manager has come up here to do.

Wilson also, according to lots of fans online, made a sly but not-so-subtle dig at his old gaffer when referring to how good training under Howe was: 'We're obviously training with a lot more intensity now.' Okay, maybe not so subtle. It was clear that the striker was keen to emphasise that Howe took no prisoners from day one, that he was keen to get down to business straightaway and that the team's fitness was probably lacking somewhat under the old boss. 'The test that we did, the bleep test, was just a six-minute one, but that was to gauge where our fitness levels are.'

Still, Wilson was also keen to address the point that any player objections to the new training regime or any teething spats would be firmly dealt with:

> He'll clamp down on any discipline and anything that needs to be done. He'll demand high standards and professionalism – all the things that you need to be to compete in the Premier League week-in, week-out. If we have that it will ultimately bring a togetherness. That's the environment they're trying to create here. You go on to the pitch and you're running for each other, working for the manager and the team-mates. It's not just each individual. We're a team, a club and all United together.

Expectations were high for Saturday's match against Brentford, and Wilson knew their training was preparing them for a different style of play:

> To play a certain style of play you have to cope with the demands of that training. And we want to play attacking football. To do that, you need to train this way [intensely], and to train that way you have to improve your fitness levels. For us, this has been a good time now to get some more high-speed runs into our legs and more intensity into our legs. Hopefully that will stand us in good stead for when the games start coming thick and fast.

My husband was in agreement.

> Chris: A new manager always has a bit of a positive impact on the team. But when Howe, who came with all this previous history of an attacking style of play, well, that's what we wanted the boys to do too.

It must have been a strange time for the Newcastle squad. In the weeks after the takeover, losing their current manager and then having these big names being flung around, you wonder what that did for camp mentality. For example, what are they told? Do they read all the rumours? Do they have any insider info? Wilson confirmed:

> In football, you try to focus on your job but you do hear people talking about different managers coming in or getting messages from people. But you try to focus on your job. Right now, though, the new owners see him as the perfect fit and it's been a great week. The transition has been great with the new manager.

'Eddie is a mastermind, a genius, a tactician,' confirms Josh Clarke, better known as @Geordie_josh on Instagram. But

Howe wasn't complacent about how well the training was going. His mind was on the job ahead. In an interview with the BBC at the start of his tenure, it was clear he didn't have a long-term plan but instead was keen to take things one day at a time. Not slowly, not tentatively, just day by day, match by match:

> It's going to take a lot of hard work instilling what we want in the players. Their application so far has been hugely impressive but we're going to need that to be consistent for us to get there. All we can do, and I know it's a cliche, is to look on the horizon and to the next game. Try to win that and then try to prepare better for the next game after that. The task ahead is huge. I'm under no illusions and I'm not saying it's going to be easy. We have a very difficult fixture list ahead, and in December.

And then Covid struck. Ironically, a few days before the Brentford game, Eddie joked that the reason for his gravelly, near-lost voice was that he'd been shouting at his players for the past two weeks. But a positive test the day before the match during a routine testing by the club revealed Covid to be the culprit and it was confirmed that he'd miss his very first match in charge of his new team.

And the headlines would again focus not on the football but on the drama from the club – five points from safety and 19th in the Premier League, and now the new man in charge won't even be there to see his first game. But nothing, not even the lingering force of the pandemic, would dent his focus on the job. He'd already organised, in case of such an eventuality, a plan ensuring that he'd FaceTime each player before the game and be in constant communication with his backroom staff in the shape of assistant head coaches Jason Tindall and Graeme Jones. There was no lost focus, it was all about getting the job done. And there was no looking further than that first game.

> We're having to implement our philosophy in a gradual manner so the players aren't overloaded, but the basic fundamentals of how we want to play, of our core principles. I'd like to think you'll see that against Brentford. I'd like to think you'll see a Newcastle team playing in the way I want them to; a way that also befits what Newcastle supporters want to see as well. How quickly can we get there? We'll see. But I'd like to think you'll see a team doing the city proud.

Due to the UK Government guidance that meant anyone with a positive test must isolate at home for ten days, not only would Howe miss this first match against Brentford but also potentially Newcastle's league fixture at Arsenal on 27 November. It wasn't an ideal start but Howe, who experienced no symptoms and looked a picture of health during a media address, and who'd been double vaccinated, knew he'd worked the players hard the past couple of weeks and that they were ready. Howe told the press conference, which he conducted via Zoom on Friday morning:

> I'm very disappointed that I won't be there with you all at St James' Park tomorrow. But it's incredibly important I follow the guidelines and self-isolate. I'd like to reassure everyone I feel fine, and while this is unwelcome news for me, I know it hasn't derailed our preparations for an important game.

Ever the positive leader, he was keen to stress how him not being on the sidelines for his first game wasn't going to be the big deal that the press were making it out to be:

> I have been, and will be, in constant communication with my coaching team and the players, both tomorrow and during the week, and I know they'll be giving everything on and off the pitch.

It's interesting to note that at this point in Howe's very initial journey into the Tyneside training ground he was already indicating that he intended to rebuild Newcastle United around midfielder Jonjo Shelvey and to unlock the ability that the Brazilian forward Joelinton had displayed at Hoffenheim. The latter, since moving to Tyneside in the summer, had been struggling horribly:

> Joelinton can be a huge player for us. From what I've seen in training he's got very, very good feet, he's very good technically and he's intelligent. Unlocking that talent and ability and playing him in the right position are things I'm assessing, but he's got a big part in our future here.

Jonjo, signed by Steve McClaren, had spent significant periods of his St James' Park career on the sidelines after being dropped fairly consistently by Rafa Benítez and Steve Bruce. But Howe believed he could be a key player to help move the team away from a defensive, counter-attacking side to a much more front-foot, possession-based team:

> I knew how good Jonjo was, having played against him and watched him many times, but when you

> actually work with him you realise he's an incredible technician. He'll be someone very important for us as the season develops and he can play all sorts of passes, long and short. In terms of our philosophy and how we want to play, he's someone who'll be very important to us.

The Brentford match, although a draw, got off to a 'winning' start. Home fans were singing Howe's name from the moment the whistle blew and it seemed that in no time at all they were grouping him with the legends of Keegan and Robson … and he wasn't even in attendance. Newcastle took an early lead, just ten minutes into the game, when Jamaal Lascelles nodded in from Matt Ritchie's corner, but it only lasted 75 seconds as Ivan Toney, a former Toon striker, took advantage of Karl Darlow's mistake to equalise and celebrate in front of the Gallowgate End. But there was still plenty of playing time left in the game and still another four goals to be scored. Watching from a live feed, Howe then saw Brentford take the lead after 31 minutes when Sergi Canós's back-post cross found Rico Henry, who volleyed a shot past Darlow. But there was only an eight-minute wait before another goal, and Joelinton, to the delight of the Toon Army, levelled the scores and curled in his first goal of the season.

In the 61st minute Brentford went ahead once more when substitute Frank Onyeka's shot was deflected past Darlow via Lascelles for a frustrating own goal. It was then that Howe decided to bring on Ryan Fraser, which proved to be a wise decision when he crossed for Allan Saint-Maximin's equaliser. 'At 3-2 down we had a decision to make and, in dialogue with Ed, those subs we made were jointly done,' said Tindall, having had a fairly unique first game without the boss next to him pitch-side. 'But Ed has to take a lot of credit for that, he's the manager and he makes the final call. Bringing on Ryan Fraser certainly made the difference for us and he played his part in the third goal for Maxi.'

Newcastle had earned themselves a point with the draw but they were still without a win. To a sellout crowd they'd conceded three goals and, crushingly, due to other results, they now found themselves in 20th position in the table. This was the worst start to a league campaign they'd ever faced. But Geordies never say die, and what came out of that first game of Howe in charge was both a sense of monumental work that had to be done, but also, dare we say, hope. They played attacking football, they didn't seem demoralised and Howe wasn't afraid to make changes to alter the dynamic of the game. Fabian Schär, Joe Willock and Joelinton replaced Emil Krafth, Isaac Hayden and Miguel Almirón from the team that had started the 1-1 draw at Brighton.

Seven days later came an away game at Arsenal, for which Eddie Howe made an unexpected return to the technical area after returning a negative Covid-19 test. Having been self-isolating in his hotel room since he tested positive, he'd be on the touchline at the Emirates. Howe hadn't been at the training ground in the run-up to the match, but assistant Jason Tindall confirmed that the head coach had been heavily involved, had been speaking to players over the phone and had been in touch with him and the other coaches up to six times a day – before and after training and then in the evening to plan for the following day. Sessions were all recorded from various angles and Howe had reviewed them, given his feedback and spoken to some players over the phone. Tindall told reporters on Zoom:

> Every team wants their manager, their leader, on the sideline. It's the person they look to for guidance, instruction and comfort, so it's really important for the football club that Ed's there. I'm not surprised because I know Eddie very well. Ed's a hands-on manager, a hands-on coach. He wants to be involved and he has been involved in all the preparation this week so we've been in constant dialogue to deliver what the manager wants us to deliver in preparation for the Arsenal game. Sometimes I do tell him he just needs to relax and rest, but it's not the character of Eddie, that's for sure.

There was no doubt in the mind of Tindall that having Howe in the dugout would have a huge impact for the team mentality: 'For the players to see the manager there will be a huge lift for them.'

And it was no surprise to learn that Howe loves nothing more than being a 'tracksuit manager', as he told *The Chronicle*:

> I think being in a tracksuit is another example that I'm not too far away from them and I'm supporting them. I know it might sound quite strange but I don't want to be seen as different to them. We're all as one. It's a way of staying close to them and I always want that closeness with my players on matchdays. That's why I never really sit down. I'm always at the front because I want my players to know that I'm with them in every moment. Whether it's good, bad or we've scored a goal or conceded a goal, I'm at the front and leading with them.

Playing the Gunners is a traditionally tricky match and this was no different. Arsenal had won their past ten home games against Newcastle in all competitions and had never lost a Premier League home game against a team sitting bottom of the table. Meanwhile, Newcastle were also creating statistics – but of the more negative kind – by being a team on the longest-ever winless run from the start of a league season.

Only one side has ever stayed up in the Premier League after failing to win their opening 13 games: Derby County in 2000/01.

Not that Howe would have identified this match as an opportunity to pick up points, of course. Even with their leader with them and leading the charge, Newcastle failed to score and lost 2-0, but, perhaps more frustratingly, were going into their next game against Norwich City without captain Jamaal Lascelles and Matt Ritchie, both suspended. The Canaries were coming to St James' Park just three days after the Arsenal game and the pressure was on. The press, the fans and most of the country determined this to be a 'must-win game' for United. Eddie was optimistic in the (short) run-up to the game as pressure was equally on Norwich, who occupied 19th position in the table. He was also excited to be in the dugout for his first game at St James' and believed that a win, the first of the 2021/22 campaign, was on the cards:

> I loved coming to St James' Park as an opposition manager and thought it was a fantastic arena to watch football in, sampling the atmosphere. To have the home supporters with us will be an amazing, unique experience and one I can't wait to sample.

Not even the thought of being without two prominent members of his squad dampened his enthusiasm for the upcoming match, signalling him to be a manager who saw potential in all his players:

> The two suspensions are going to be big misses for us with the experience they have but I don't think there's any fresh injuries from Saturday and there's going to be opportunities. When you have suspensions or injuries, it's a disappointment for those players involved but an opportunity for someone else, which is good for us to see the squad. I'm confident whoever comes in will give a very good account of themselves for the team. We know it's going to be a really tough game. We cannot underestimate Norwich in any way. Any Premier League game is incredibly tough to win so we know we'll have to be at our very best.

Impressed by his side's attacking form, particularly against Brentford, Howe was keen to reiterate that his team, the team he'd been working with for just shy of one month, were already a different team to the one he inherited:

> Going back to our last home game, the amount of chances we created with over 20 shots, we looked a good attacking threat. There were moments the other way that weren't so stable but I saw enough from it as an attacking side to know we can create and score goals and I saw the same at Arsenal. We created enough in the game away from home against a really tough opponent to know that we'll be in games from an attacking perspective. I thought there were positive signs, albeit in defeat. We know we

> can't keep saying that and have to turn these small margins that are costing us games the other way, but I'm sure we can do it.

Howe also knew, whatever the result in the Norwich City game, his team would be facing Burnley, a fellow relegation rival, just four days later. It was a busy time for Newcastle and one during which they needed to pick up points. Preferably get that much-sought-after first win. But Eddie didn't want to get ahead of himself:

> It's been a very busy time, with three games in a week coming up, and we're looking forward to the challenges that we face this week. We're aware how important these games are but I think it's a dangerous thing to look too far ahead. Firstly, I'm looking at training today and then, of course, tomorrow's game. It's always a step-by-step process. The minute you start looking too far ahead, you can take your eye off the priorities. The priorities right now are the players and preparing them as best we can for the next game.

But, ten Magpies do not a team make. Against Norwich, the sending off of Ciaran Clark after nine minutes for a foul on Pukki didn't impress the St James' Park crowd. Callum Wilson was named Newcastle captain in the absence of the suspended Lascelles, and his penalty gave a glimmer of hope, but the match ended 1-1.

I asked my son about what he thought of Howe at this stage of the game, as it were, and, in brutally honest 11-year-old fashion, he told it to me straight:

> Henry: I was a bit nervous of him to start with, Mum, because you would be, wouldn't you? But after the first game I knew he would be a winner as he was getting our players to move around – he moved Joelinton from up front to midfield in the Norwich game and he's a much better player in this position. He's strong, a powerhouse, and more comfortable where he is there.

It was a good point. And one that the press and fans in their thousands agreed with. A win against Norwich might have bypassed the Magpies once again (albeit through a 79th-minute equaliser rather than a complete whitewash) but the match provided something of a revelation for a £40m signing who wasn't having the best start to his Tyneside career.

Joelinton arrived at Newcastle in the summer of 2019 from Hoffenheim, after Rafa Benítez had left the club and Steve Bruce was appointed as his replacement. Bruce and the coaching team saw him as Salomón Rondón's successor and handed him the iconic No.9 shirt. But there ends the fairy tale. It took the Brazilian 26 games and 39 shots to score his first goal and he only managed to add five more to his tally across his first two seasons at Newcastle. To say he was fast becoming the scapegoat for the lack of success was an understatement. But all that changed after the Norwich City game on 30 November. Not because he suddenly put his scoring boots on (they'd gone missing somewhere in the Tyne) but because he was no longer expected to score. His focus was elsewhere on the pitch and that position shift proved to be dynamite. Howe reflected on the change:

> When we initially came in we thought Joelinton would play as a number ten, a second striker. But we went down to ten men against Norwich and reshuffled and played him as an eight, and he was brilliant defensively. He has a tactical understanding and his attitude, work rate and energy are top level. His technique and ability to find space and control the ball in tight areas is of the highest level. I love the lad to bits.

It was like a fire had been lit and the Brazilian powerhouse had come home. Howe had recognised his potential from the very first training session, something that the previous managers had failed to see. But in typical self-deprecating style, he refused to take credit for this new midfield machine, as he told *The Athletic*:

> I remember seeing him in our first training session and thinking, wow, what a player he is. I didn't know too much about what had happened to him here, but that initial impression was of an outstanding talent who also seemed like a really good guy. My opinion hasn't changed. When you see a player do well – and improve dramatically in Joe's case – it gives you a great source of satisfaction, but the credit lies with him.

But it was Howe who was credited with releasing the player from his up-front prison and giving him the space to exert his influence in the middle of the pitch. It was a move that was to see him become one of Newcastle's best defensive and attacking players all in one – registering more interceptions, clearances and tackles than Newcastle's forwards in the 2021/22 campaign.

'The moment Joelinton moved to central midfield was the moment he started playing football,' recalled James. 'He was playing in his best position. He has incredible power and terrific pace.'

> Chris: I remember watching Joelinton playing midfield and thinking, *When did he get so good?* He had an outstanding midfield performance against Norwich and after that seemed to get better and better. He had everything. It was like watching a totally different person because, let's face it, he was shit as a centre-forward, but now he's one of Newcastle's best players.

It's not just fans who are keen to celebrate the player. His central midfield partner in crime Sean Longstaff is keen for the world and its wife to know that the bad press Joelinton received before his positional move was unfair:

> We know how good Joelinton is and the disrespect he gets is a disgrace. Every day in training he's the best player and if you get him on your team in training you're buzzing because you'll always win. He's shown since the manager came in what he's like and everyone at the club rates him so highly. The noise from outside is so disrespectful and if you watch him enough you see how good he is. I'm so happy for him and proud of him.

And the man himself?

It seemed that Howe had instilled in him a confidence that had been missing the past couple of years. 'It's a new position for me,' Joelinton confirmed. 'I try to give everything for the team and I understand what the manager is asking from me on the pitch.'

He wasn't the only player that the gaffer saw as hidden talent, and Howe was keen to share how in those early days he went about getting the best out of Allan Saint-Maximin too:

> With someone like Allan, what I've tried to do is understand how he thinks, what he needs to be the best he can be and I work backwards from that point. And that's where I say being able to control my emotions well helps in those situations. You put that to one side and think, *What does he need to help him?* I've been able to condition my brain to think that way.

Our Geordie neighbour has the final word.

> Sharon: Eddie is an intelligent coach and empathetic across all areas of the game, as I can see. Obviously I'm biased but as a football fan I think he comes across as committed and invested in all and everything at the club.

Chapter 5

Starting as We Mean to Go On

'Anyone can support a team that is winning – it takes no courage. But to stand behind a team when it is down and really needs you, that takes a lot of courage.'

Bart Starr

'IT'S REALLY depressing hearing fans who are passionate about the club, love the city, but haven't got the one thing that all fans need: hope. You have to have hope, and Newcastle haven't had it.' Gary Neville spoke these words back in September 2021 as Newcastle were about to play Leeds United. It was the sixth game in which they hadn't won. And that losing streak wasn't going to end for another three months.

November 2021 was one heck of a month for Newcastle. For all the excitement sparked and the hope it ignited, for all the talk that an exciting new era had begun at one of English football's great underachievers, nothing really changed. Steve Bruce had been sacked, Eddie Howe had been appointed and still Newcastle couldn't win. Leads were taken, leads were lost and the Magpies were bottom of the table and in danger of being cut adrift long before the new owners got to spend any money in the January transfer window. Howe had brought hope and excitement to the club and its loyal supporters but, as the first month of his tenure drew to a close, it was time to assess the impact of the managerial change at St James' Park.

His influence on the team was apparent. The players seemed to have bought into his philosophy and style of play, displaying a cohesion and unity that had been lacking in the early stages of the season. Off the pitch, Howe had fostered a positive and harmonious atmosphere within the squad.

Players spoke glowingly about the new manager's approach, citing his communication skills and ability to instil confidence and belief in the team. The unity and camaraderie within the squad were palpable, with a sense of togetherness and purpose driving the team forward. And yet, with no win to their name since the start of the season, Howe's job wasn't to overhaul the team in his first season as manager, it was to do enough tweaking to convert the frustrated draws into wins, to get enough points to keep Newcastle in the Premier League.

Howe remained pragmatic in his assessment of the lack of wins after the Norwich match, acknowledging the need for further development and refinement in certain areas of the team:

> We know we need wins, draws aren't going to be enough. But I think all you can do in every game is give your all, and I think you saw a group of players who gave that. I couldn't ask any more of those players who committed to the task ahead so I have to be very proud and pleased with them.

Recording their first win of the season wouldn't just make the Premier League table look better for them – having moved from 19th to 20th for the last ten games was getting a little tiresome – it would also dramatically improve the squad's mentality.

As Neville alluded to, hope can be a cruel emotion, but losing is an equally challenging experience for players, and it can have a significant impact on their mental health and performance. The cycle of losing creates negative thinking and self-doubt, which then has a significant impact on an athlete's performance and ability to bounce back. According to sports psychologist Amy Goldstaff, when athletes only focus on their failures it leads to defeat in their minds before they've even taken to the pitch. And then, if they're losing in a game, they make sloppy mistakes and believe their situation is hopeless because they're only used to that feeling of loss:

> Stress and anxiety are common experiences for players, particularly in high-pressure situations such as big cup games or competitions but it's worse if they have experienced a run of draws and losses. They forget what winning feels like and so they 'get used' to the feeling of failure. This means that they lose their 'comeback' mindset, they don't believe there is any point in fighting for the ball in the hopes of coming back from behind, they just accept what they believe to be their 'fate'.

Of course, when it comes to professional football teams, there's an army of psychologists and coaching staff to ensure that every game has a positive focus and that if athletes are stressed or anxious, they don't experience physical symptoms such as tension, headaches and increased heart rates, which can all impact their performance during a match.

Dan Abrahams, who has been a sports psychologist for over ten years and has previously worked for Queens Park Rangers, Derby County and the England rugby union team, understands the impact the individual player's mentality has on the team as well as the knock-on effect on the managers, the coaching staff and the fans. He said, in an online interview in 2017:

> Just as they need to be able to compete when they're 60–80 per cent fit, it's possible for players to compete effectively even when you're not confident. Managers get so annoyed, not at the 6/10 or the 7/10 performance but at the 4/10 performance. If you do make a few bad passes, you do give the ball away, you do miss a chance on goal, you do concede a soft goal, get that body language back up, impose yourself, stay on your toes no matter what, stay lively – that's a really important thing. It doesn't make you man of the match but it turns a 6/10 into a 7/10 and a 7/10 into an 8/10.

Abrahams also talked about the players being able to put things into perspective, making sure they can remember what winning feels like and that it's not an alien concept, it's a memory they can draw upon. From a mentality point of view, the best footballers are the ones that are constantly able to improve themselves from both a physical and mental point of view – and they can draw on their winning experiences when they need to:

> I say to players all of the time, champions are champions because they're really good at remembering themselves at their best – their best games, best moments and remembering it in detail, like the runs they made, the movement they had, the passes they make and what that feels like so they kind of have a rich sensory experience.

By all accounts, developing strategies for coping with losing or drawing game after game and the pressure that Newcastle were under now that the club had new owners and a new manager would have been key to them focusing on a win. Even players like Wilson, who'd been vocal before (at length) about fitness, believed the old regime was still hindering their performance, saying: 'We weren't fit enough and we weren't in the right place. The pre-season is massive for the way it sets you up for the season.' It was a sentiment echoed by my father-in-law.

> Grampy: Under Bruce, no one was training as they should. A lot of players were having private training because they knew what they were getting from the club wasn't enough. Howe made them train and made them train well and that was the first thing you noticed under his leadership; we could last 90 minutes whereas we couldn't before. We'd always, around the 70-minute mark, more or less have had it. And then players who hadn't been great before were suddenly there and performing for Howe and having a phenomenal impact on the pitch. I believe that if Joelinton had come under Eddie Howe from the word go it would have been different. But he came under Steve Bruce and he couldn't improve

> a world-class player – if anything he'd bring them down to a lower level.

And then, of course, you add in the historical weight of Newcastle's situation – that the media like to talk about, ask about and report about on repeat – the fact that no Premier League club had ever managed to avoid relegation after a start to the season as bad as Newcastle's.

But there was one person who hadn't given up and wouldn't give up. Howe wasn't just a motivator, he was an unruffled voice, a calm among the dramatic pundits who liked to scream about Newcastle's predicted demise. He was the whisper of composure:

> I was always very calm – that's my personality. If there's a problem, then I'll try to go away and fix it and work to find solutions, not really panicking or reacting adversely.

He hasn't changed. For all the talk of flamboyant managers and A-list gaffers from La Liga, Chelsea, etc., it's arguably Howe's coolness that has guided the club through one of its toughest times to date.

> I'm very much a thinker, so I was very calm and I always believed. I always believed in the players – and that was regardless of the transfer window – I always believed that we could stay in the division. I said that many times and I don't say it if I don't believe it. I believe you can do special things on the training ground with players, you can improve players to a level that they don't think they're capable of. I still feel we have a long way to go in that respect, but the

> training ground work is what I love and that's what we'll really be focusing on for pre-season.

Poor performance and failure can, of course, have a significant impact on fans, which in turn can have an effect on the team. Remembering that the Toon Army are the best fans in the world and show support no matter what, even they were getting to a point of defeat. And having gone from such a high only a few months previously during the takeover, this wasn't the fairy tale beginning they were desperate for.

> Chris: I remember just thinking, *please just find the back of the net, please keep a lead.* But even I found that I was losing interest in the games. I just wasn't following the team much after a while, as the assumption was that Newcastle would just lose.

And while it's most notably athletes whose experience of frequent losses or poor performances can result in feelings of shame, embarrassment and disappointment, which can lead to a decrease in motivation and self-confidence, it also has a strong knock-on effect with fans.

> Alan: It felt like there was no light at the end of the tunnel. It looked like we were never going to experience a win.

And for those who remembered the relegation days, it just brought back bad memories.

> Rob: I just thought, *Here we go again, we're going to get relegated, that's that.*

> Sarah: Despite lining up for games where we knew we were the better side, we either couldn't hang on to a lead or we'd just get beat. We lost a belief in ourselves that we'd ever get a win. And then instead of hoping for a win, you find yourself desperately clinging on for a draw. How is that even right?! That you just pray for a draw because you've given up hoping for a win and a draw is a softer blow than a loss.

Of course, when poor results begin to snowball, pressure then mounts, and it's an extremely tough cycle to break. But break it they did. At the 15th time of asking. On the fourth day of Christmas (well, December), Newcastle Football Club gave to me, a win (at last!) against Burn-ley.

This victory was needed. It wasn't just about three points to close the gap on the teams above them, but to give Newcastle their long-awaited 'new era' lift-off. Of course, it wasn't without drama, and any nervous fingernail chewers would have been left without even a slither in the final ten minutes, which were both torturous and stressful. But for the first time in what felt like an eternity (well, since May), Newcastle won – and came away with a clean sheet.

It didn't get off to a cohesive start. St James' Park roared as the players came out on to the pitch and fans kept up the noise as the whistle blew, but Newcastle were slow in their response to the support. With Burnley as fellow relegation rivals, it seemed Newcastle were hesitant. They didn't want to make a mistake, and this saw them passing slowly, timidly and deliberately. It wasn't a game plan that was getting them anywhere and the fans voiced their disapproval. 'I remember shouting in frustration at the players to wake up,' recalls Dan. 'I wasn't the only one. There was a real sense in the stadium that what we were seeing wasn't enough and the fans were demanding more. We definitely deserved to see more!'

Whether it was the fans being unusually angrily vocal or that Burnley nearly went ahead when Gudmundsson's shot hit the post, Newcastle players realised they needed to start coming alive. It was like they agreed with the fans, enough was enough.

After 20 minutes of slow, mediocre play, Callum Wilson's goal gave the stadium something to cheer about. It eased the tension, liberating Newcastle's players, and they pushed forward for the second goal that would give them breathing space. It didn't come. Almirón either couldn't hit the target or, when he did, his shot was diverted away from the top corner by a Burnley head.

With an hour played, Newcastle's lead remained a slender one, and a defence that hadn't kept a clean sheet all season was always in danger of calamity. Burnley weren't offering much of an attacking threat at this stage but they were holding their defensive line. Newcastle had been in this winning position before, but so far this season had let it slip away. This was a real test of nerves. As the clock crept towards full time, the tension was unbearable. Suddenly, in the last ten minutes, Burnley decided to push for an equaliser and Newcastle, now looking tired, were in danger of yet again losing the lead.

> Chris: I thought time was going backwards. I just wanted the ref to blow the whistle. It was excruciating!

Newcastle abandoned any thought of adding to their lead and the sole focus was to defend their one-goal advantage. And they did. When the final whistle blew, tens of thousands of eyes looked to the heavens as the relief swelled through the hearts of the home crowd. The noise that followed was so deafening that it was heard across the city – it was a deep, belly roar and it filled the stadium at the realisation that they'd won their first game and the celebrations could begin. Around the country, the cheers in the pubs, clubs and homes were the same. It was a clashing of pure relief, the chance to let out a breath that many had been holding, and then there was time to celebrate not just a win but a clean sheet.

As the fans cheered and sang and the players and coaching staff received the applause and whipped up the euphoria inside the stadium another notch, it was difficult not to believe that this was the start of something. Surely it was the start of something … But ever the realist, Eddie was the calming voice and the reminder that it was and always will be one match at a time. It had taken him four games to see a success as their manager and he knew he couldn't go another four games until the next one if they wanted to climb out of the relegation zone.

Howe said, when asked about how he felt after his first win as manager of the club:

> Mixture of emotions really. Definite relief. Very proud of the team. It was a very difficult game physically, as it always is against Burnley, but I thought we defended very, very well today. We took a lot of positives from the midweek game against Norwich and I think, to a man, really, really stepped up again defensively. We started the game quite slowly – first 20 minutes was a bit disappointing – but once we scored, there were spells in the second half where I thought we were excellent. We had to hang on at the end. It was a nervy end to the match.

Eddie knew the home crowd had played a big part in this victory. Very few clubs build such a momentum as efficiently as this when the synergy between the team and supporters are this powerful and it didn't go unnoticed to Howe:

> The relationship we've quickly built with the supporters has been a really special one. I thought they were absolutely magnificent today for the club – I can't thank them enough and it's just an amazing feeling to get that first win for them as a big thank you for everything they've given to me and the team the last few weeks. We knew how desperate they were for that first victory, we all were, but to get it was an amazing feeling. The reaction at the end, the scenes with the players, that can only galvanise us to hopefully move forward positively.

While that win was a joyous occasion, Newcastle knew their fixtures over the festive period weren't going to be gift-wrapped, with games against Leicester, Liverpool, Manchester City and Manchester United across the final month of the year.

While spirits were lifted that they'd finally got a positive result after their winless streak, an away game against Leicester was soon to scupper the momentum. Initially there was a potential upset on the cards when Almirón fired into the side netting, unnerving an uncertain Leicester defence. But it was not to be. Newcastle lost 4-0 in what Howe called a scoreline that was 'not reflective' of how they'd played. 'Statistics show us that, and my gut feeling tells me that, but we have to regroup very quickly,' he said. And that wasn't an understatement, as in the next seven days they had to face Liverpool at Anfield before hosting Manchester City on 19 December, the final game before Christmas.

Again, against Liverpool, early momentum was on their side. This was a team that had tasted victory and liked it. And it was a brilliant start. Howe had decided to rest top scorer Wilson, and Miguel Almirón and Joe Willock, opting for a 4-5-1 formation, seeking to counter-attack at pace. It was a tactic that worked. Just eight minutes into the game Jonjo Shelvey scored a magnificent goal – even if it came from Thiago's mistake. Who cared? The Toon Army were elated and the midfielder sprinted the length of the pitch to celebrate with his fans. It was his first goal since February. They had another chance to score and raise the roof at the away end but, in the end, they once more showed their defensive fragility by losing two goals in quick succession and then struggled to make many clear-cut opportunities to draw level. They did, though, have a penalty appeal waved away when they believed Ryan Fraser was brought down by Alexander-Arnold.

Newcastle firmed up in the second half, however, and Howe's tactics looked as if they might yield a point, before Alexander-Arnold's strike took the game away from the visitors. It was a 3-1 defeat but there were a lot of positives to take from it. Howe couldn't fault his players, who were playing with the big boys and were competing again – albeit not with positive results, but he was less impressed with the referee and the decision not to stop the game before Jota equalised in the 21st minute:

> We really competed, the lads gave everything to the game. We had a plan and scored a great goal. The game turns on a decision I can't understand. I can't

> believe Mike Dean hasn't stopped the game. Isaac Hayden was holding his head and we had two players down. It shows how goals change games. The game changes on that incident and the crowd gets behind them. We're on the wrong end of the 50-50 calls at the moment.

But they had to regroup as just three days later they were hosting Manchester City. And Pep Guardiola's fans were keen to remind the Toon that, for all Newcastle's riches, money couldn't buy them points in the Premier League. 'All that money and you're going down' came the chant from the upper Leazes Stand. Although in fairness, this was quite possibly in response to the roars of 'We're richer than you!' from the Gallowgate End.

They had a point. Newcastle United were significantly richer than Man City but they weren't in the league of the Citizens. After just five minutes Newcastle went behind and then followed three more goals by the visitors. The 4-0 defeat meant that they went into Christmas firmly in relegation trouble. But there was no one more positive than Howe:

> To play them with two days' less recovery and the physical efforts of the players was extraordinary after the efforts against Liverpool. There was a good feeling about the team, a good structure and good moments in the match. We're heading in the right direction but a long way to go. We gave ourselves a mountain to climb with the goal we conceded and we conceded a poor second goal. But it's a really strange game because the results look bleak for us, the reality of the game feels very different.

The press weren't quite as optimistic, as Richard Harris, a sports journalist, showed:

> It is looking more and more like the decision to sack Steve Bruce and bring in Eddie Howe has backfired. Bruce was largely undermined by injuries to key players. Howe isn't noted for his ability to organise the defence, and boy does it show. If Newcastle are relegated the new owners will need to look at themselves and accept they messed up big time. Of course they could buy a £200 million new team next week so I may be proved wrong.

It was a keen observation. And one felt keenly by my father-in-law.

> Grampy: We had so many bad years previously, it was becoming the norm that we weren't going to win. That's not right, is it? And at that time, Howe was still a bit of unknown to the majority of us. We were wondering if he was the right man to stop this losing streak. And it certainly didn't seem like it at first.

It was January soon and the transfer window would be wide open. This meant the purse strings could finally be opened. But first there was a home match against the other Manchester club as St James' Park welcomed the Red Devils on to the pitch on 27 December.

Instead of following the supposed script and pressing Newcastle into submission, Rangnick's disjointed team were frequently pulled apart by Allan Saint-Maximin's attacking manoeuvres and Joelinton's midfield excellence. It was Saint-Maximin's seventh-minute goal that raised the roof at St James', but there was so long left of the game that the defence had a lot of work to do to maintain the lead. And it was a lead they managed to keep until the 71st minute, when Edinson Cavani scored the equaliser. But, strangely, even the draw couldn't dent the optimistic feeling that surged from the home crowd. It wasn't a victory, but the new year was only a matter of days away and for the majority of home fans who left the stands that afternoon there was still hope that relegation could be avoided.

Results may have disappointed them since Howe had succeeded Steve Bruce but the newcomer's man management had certainly brought the best out of an apparently reinvented Joelinton. And Howe was still full of gratitude for his team:

> I can't praise the players enough. It was an excellent performance. I'm really pleased. We deserved to win and you're left with the horrible feeling of not getting what you deserve. We gave a lot to the match physically and we had some really good moments. Allan Saint-Maximin at the start of the second half was a good chance. Jacob Murphy hit the post and Miguel Almirón's shot looked like it was in. It's good to talk about these moments. There have been games where we haven't created.
>
> Joelinton was very good today, his defensive understanding in that position is incredible. His attitude, work rate and energy are top level. His technique and ability to find space and control the ball in tight areas is of the highest level. I love the lad to bits. I'm really glad he's performing so well. We're capable of beating anybody. We proved that

> today. I thought we all performed today. That's got to be the standard we've set ourselves. We can be a force to be reckoned with.

And a force they were about to become.

Chapter 6

January Sales

'Magpie, n.: A bird whose thievish disposition suggested to someone that it might be taught to talk.'

Ambrose Bierce

NEW YEAR, new start and the PIF purse was open. Howe was keen to share the news the owners were focused on, who they wanted and why:

> We have targets we've identified between myself, the coaching team and the recruitment team and we have a big body of people working on the club's behalf to try and find a way to strengthen the squad.

It was an exciting time for fans. Never before had so much money been available to spend and with so many opportunities.

'It was like taking a kid into a sweet shop,' said Barney. 'It was like we could literally look at all the best players across all the best teams and be, like, "I want that one!"'

Kicking off the sweet-shop haul was England right-back Kieran Trippier. He was a huge signing – and a big statement from the club, arriving from Atlético Madrid for £12m plus add-ons. Interestingly, when the transfer window was opened two years later in 2024, Bayern Munich were keen to snap up the defender, which would have made him one of the club's original best signings. Howe had gone to watch Atlético train a few months before and had spent a couple of days with Tripps:

> We'd got talking about his future and coming back to England was something on his mind. As soon as I got the job, it was straightaway, 'Right, Kieran, let's speak to him and see.' The thing I loved about his attitude was something very similar to Bruno [a signing made a little later, be patient, pet]; there were no relegation or escape clauses, all-in, desperate to come, wanted to pull on the black-and-white shirt. That was so refreshing. Getting the right characters in like that, people who just wanted to fight and had no way out, is so powerful.

Trippier was excited about coming to join the Toon squad and was keen to stress that his move was due to wanting a challenge rather than for financial gain:

> I'm aware there's a lot of work ahead of us but I know the demands of Premier League well and I know what an amazing club this is with very talented players. I can't wait to get started and I'm excited to step out at St James' Park as a Newcastle player. If people say it's about money, then everybody's entitled to their own opinion, but I know my reasons why and that's not one of them.

Howe was equally keen to stress that the status of the club and the excitement of playing for Newcastle was the reason Trippier signed:

> It's a sign that the club has a huge pull – and I'm not talking financial here. Kieran hasn't come for the financial benefits of the contract. He's come for the club and for the challenge that the team faces at the current time, but also the longer-term vision, so I think that's a massive thing for the football club. Hopefully, with his signing, other players around the world will potentially look at that and share his dream and his vision for what he sees.

My son was a happy boy:

> Henry: I'd watched Trippier play for England so I was so happy when he was our first signing. I knew he would fit right in with the team.

Howe was confident of more signings in the transfer window but was keen to stress that things might not be as easy as the outside world and fans might think:

> We're in the hands of clubs selling players, we're in the hands of agents and players wanting to come. There are no guarantees. It might sound simple from the outside; it's very, very different when you're on the inside, so I'm confident, but there are no promises. Character is a huge part of what we do in recruitment.

It was again a good reminder from the level-headed man in charge for everyone not to get too excited. Just like your dad would tell you to think carefully about what you want to buy in the sweet shop.

> Rob: I was dead excited about Trippier. But then, I was excited about all the players we were going to get!

> Grampy: Everyone was expecting top-quality players to come in, that was the talk on the fans forums. Then it became obvious the FFP [Financial Fair Play], that started getting mentioned by the club to make sure the fans were aware of what that meant. Most of us wouldn't have known about Fair Play or what it was, as it didn't affect us under Ashley. We always ran a profit under Ashley but we didn't have a loss or negative figures, so we were never going to breach Fair Play because we never spent any money. Simple as that. We knew that the new owners had wealth, but they were a company, there was talk of them wanting the club to do well but there was no proof. I knew Trippier, but he was 31 years old and I thought, *You've got to be doing better.* Then I saw him play and I knew different. I don't think we'd seen anything like him before at Newcastle and he was terrific.

On 13 January, Tyneside was buzzing again with the news that Burnley player Chris Wood had joined the squad for £25m. It was a bitter blow for the Clarets, Newcastle's fellow relegation rivals, but it was clear Howe wanted some attacking reinforcements with Wilson being out injured, and he was impressed with Wood's scoring record:

> Chris is an important signing for us at a crucial time and I'm very pleased we've been able to move

> quickly and bring him here. He's a very dangerous attacking threat, has a physicality and character that I really like, and he has vast experience in the Premier League. He'll be a great fit for us.

While poor Burnley would feel the loss after losing their key striker – they were indeed relegated that season – Wood told us a lot about his character and his loyalty as a player and a person when he joined the Toon:

> This is a massive opportunity and club, and something I couldn't turn down. But it wasn't an easy decision. I spent four and a half great years [at Burnley]. Every single year I really enjoyed myself there. My team-mates, the staff, the club as a whole was fantastic. To be honest, I wish I'd left when Burnley were further up the league, but that's just how football is sometimes.

But the striker was also excited about the new chapter in his life and was eager to get started:

> The club and manager have been first class during this process, and I really can't wait to get on to the pitch and repay the faith they have in me, especially with a vital part of the season ahead of us.

Towards the end of the month, with their eyes still on players, Newcastle announced the big news. Arsenal had been keen to get him, Paris Saint-Germain and Manchester United had been watching him, but Bruno Guimarães was coming to the Tyne – and everyone was excited.

> Chris: To be honest, I was just happy we had money to spend. To me, though, getting a Brazilian international was exciting. Bruno was exciting.

Although his father didn't agree.

> Grampy: Bruno came in and I'd never heard of him. But thousands of fans on the forums had heard of him and everyone was excited. I trusted others at that point. He was a young player so I wondered whether he'd fit into to this English club, and he did very quickly.

Agreeing a package of £33.3m plus around £6.5m in add-ons with French club Lyon, Brazilian international Bruno Guimarães was the club's third signing. It was a huge signing but it made their intentions very clear to everyone who was watching them – they were now a force to be reckoned with and were aiming high. If only they could meet their short-term goal of avoiding relegation this season. Bruno was definitely up for the challenge:

> They [the owners] were very upfront and honest about it. They didn't disguise that the main objective and challenge was remaining in the Premier League this season. But in the seasons coming the objective is to be in the Champions League and eventually to win the Champions League.

It's testament to the strength of that initial signing that two years later Bruno signed a new contract to stay at the club for the next five years, the place where he has felt welcome since day one. 'I'm absolutely delighted. The fans have made me feel at home since my first day here,' he said, after confirming the new deal that runs until 2028. 'I feel so loved in my life.'

> Callum: Bruno has the most passion I've ever seen in our black-and-white lives since I've watched football. I can always rely on him to do us good. I hadn't heard of him when he came but he gave me great hope and it was a real confidence boost for our club.

And the rest of the city thought so too. Bruno '39' shirts (the number of his dad's taxi in Brazil) were flying off the shelves. The Brazilian was on everyone's lips. 'I've been doing my research and I know he's a big character, so I hope when he's in the dressing room he'll make everyone feel like they can step up,' recalls Jimmy. 'He's not afraid to work hard either, he's got a good engine on him.'

And for others, with one day left of the transfer window to go, it was a case of who else could they buy? Forty million pounds, the same amount as the club paid for Joelinton, was seen as a drop in the ocean with the money the new owners had but, of course, the rules on spending were tight.

'I was waiting for the £100 million-plus signings,' remembered Ben. 'I didn't really quite understand about the Financial Fair Play scheme. Mind you, we've never had to worry 'bout that either, like!'

Never ones to leave things to the last minute, on the deadline day of signings there was a double whammy of defensive strengthening as Newcastle welcomed Dan Burn and Matt Targett. It was a key move from Howe and the PIF. Although Newcastle hadn't been scoring many goals so far this season, they'd been conceding them left, right and centre. In fact, they were second only to Norwich, who'd conceded 45 goals to date. The Toon were on 43. Bringing home Dan Burn for £13m, a kid who'd been released by Newcastle at 11 years old, was a boost for the club. It was as if the magpies who had flown the nest to Brighton & Hove Albion were ready to return home.

> Alan: Bruno and Kieran were really exciting buys. But big Dan Burn, being a local lad, was great to see.

'I'm delighted to bring Dan back to the North East,' agreed Howe, which also shows an element of persistence as Brighton had previously rejected a £7m bid and then a £10m bid for Burn. Howe added:

> We've been very keen to add competition defensively and Dan fits the profile we've been looking for. He's naturally left-footed, which provides further balance to our back line, and he'll be a great addition to the group.

My father-in-law wasn't convinced, as he confessed on a windy Sunday morning as we watched my son at rugby training.

> Grampy: Dan Burn coming in, at 32 years old? I wasn't sure. Yes, of course it helped that he was born and bred in Blyth, so that made him a hit with fans, but he was nothing too inspiring for me at that time. There were lots of international players and names being thrown around, and all possibilities on forums, so I think I was swept up in the possibilities. But we had that with the names of managers too; there so many names in the mix at first but you didn't know

> who would be coming in until it was announced. I suppose Dan Burn knows what it means to represent this club and he'll be a big figure on the pitch.

Which proved to be true. At 6ft 7in, Burn was a massive presence at left-back for the team and, as a former academy player, it was a dream come true for him:

> I'm buzzing to be here. I never thought I'd be in this position, so to be a Newcastle player and to be around St James' Park, it's something I've dreamed of since I was a kid. I can't wait to step out in the shirt and to see what it feels like. From sitting in the East Stand as a kid to now, it's crazy. I'm excited to get started.

Coming back to the club he'd loved and watched and supported as a child was a huge thing. Henry and I had a conversation about this the other day. I told him that I wondered what it would mean if he ever got to play for Newcastle, and he just shook his head. 'I think you know the answer to that, Mum,' he said, rolling his eyes.

I could only imagine what it must have been like for Burn's family, all fans of the club, as they watched him being rejected from the academy at such a young age, to them now being escorted around the Tyne dressing room. Pride, disbelief, fate spring to mind. It was a sentiment that Burn understood, knowing the sacrifices his family made for him:

> It's just crazy, just to think I'm going to be running about in a Newcastle top. I don't think I've had one since I was about 13. Generations of my family have all been Newcastle fans, so I really wanted my mam and dad to be here when I was signing. They took

> us up and down the country. They came and sat and watched me on the bench at Hereford, knowing I was never getting on. They put the miles in for us.

Knowing what I know as a mum having a son live and breathe Newcastle as well as playing football with a passion and enthusiasm that I don't have in any area of my life, I can only surmise that the weight of signing for your club is probably indescribable. Burn confirmed this when talking about being dropped not long after leaving primary school:

> Me being young and naive, it probably was [a surprise] – me thinking I was a good footballer, just because I was involved. In reality, it was about right. I probably wasn't getting a game for my Sunday league team at the time, so to be thinking I could be involved in Newcastle, I was a bit deluded. But you're a kid, and you dream.

So whether he reads this or not, keep dreaming Hen.

Completing the January transfer line-up was left-back Targett, 26, who came on loan from Aston Villa until the end of this season. Howe explained the signing:

> We've gone into this transfer window with a plan to add strong competition in specific areas of the team and Matt will be a fantastic option for us on the left. He has important Premier League experience and know-how at this level, so I'm really pleased we've been able to add him to the squad.

Targett was an experienced Premier League player, having started his career at Southampton after coming through the club's academy system before going on loan to Fulham and then settling at Aston Villa in 2019:

> My family have friends here and they've always said it's a football-mad city, so to experience it and be part of it – I'm really looking forward to it. I'm coming here in good form and I'll give my all for the club. I know that the fans are very passionate and they give the team great backing. It's really exciting to be a player at this club. I'm sure everyone is keeping an eye on how Newcastle does.

So, with around £90m spent in a targeted and precise plan, was Howe pleased that the manic January was over and it was now down to business?

> It was a chaotic window. I wouldn't say we got lucky, because we made some very good decisions. We did really well, but you won't be able to deliver that long term, because you need your structures to be right. Recruitment processes have to be so good, with the competition you have around the world for players.

So, signings done, what now? Where could they pick up points? In the new year, Newcastle were set to face Watford on 15 January and Leeds seven days later. Southampton was meant to be their first fixture but it was postponed due to a Covid outbreak at the club.

It wasn't the best start. While the news of big signings was happening and bringing excitement and hope to the fans, the team still struggled for points. However, first they lost in disastrous fashion in the third round of the FA Cup at St James' Park, to a side who were in 16th position in

League One. And not only that, the Cambridge goalscorer who sealed the Toon's fate with the only goal of the game was Joe Ironside, a big Shearer fan who grew up idolising the Geordie legend.

But the positives that did come out of this game could be summed up in one word: 'Tripps.' The first signing of the January transfer window was named in the starting line-up and the chatter online was mixed. Some fans were keen to see him start, eager for his influence to set the stadium alight, make the most of the bucks the club had spent. Others weren't so sure, as they wanted Trippier rested for a while, not playing until he was needed, and it wasn't thought that an FA Cup third-round tie against a lower-tier team was the place for him to make his debut. As it turned out, it wasn't what he did during the game that proved to fans what he was made of, it was afterwards. As the final whistle blew, signalling that the Magpies had been knocked out of the FA Cup, it was Trippier who made the move to acknowledge the near-capacity ground, even though he was largely ignored. It was a clear sign that he was at the club with a purpose: he wasn't just here to play, he was here to lead by example.

According to his former PE teacher, Lee Garcka, this sort of behaviour is typical of the right-back:

> When he was at school, people looked up to him. He would try to involve everybody, in lessons and matches. If things didn't go right, he wouldn't point fingers or blame people. He'd say, 'We need to fix this, but we need to fix it together.' We were in the Year 10 cup final against a rival school who had beaten us the year before. He got everyone in a huddle before the game. I hadn't instigated it. I'd

> love to know what he said, but we won 4-1 and he scored a hat-trick.

It was clear to everyone at the game that Trippier was one of the Toon after just one game and that he understood the importance of acknowledging the support that was being shown. Support is a two-way exchange, a partnership, and he was cheered and waved as he made his way round on the lap of the pitch.

Just seven days later, Newcastle faced their first league game of 2022, at home to Watford. Saint-Maximin scored in the 49th minute, and Newcastle hung on to the lead until the 88th minute, but a second win of the season was beyond them, yet again, when Watford's Pedro headed in an equaliser. The crowd were silenced. Howe flung his water bottle down in frustration. This was their first chance to move out of the relegation zone after taking up residence there for the past 106 days. It also meant that Watford moved out of the bottom three. Heartache and frustration were felt by everyone.

The draw felt like a defeat. Remember, at this stage, the last-minute transfer window signings of Burn and Targett hadn't been made (neither had Bruno's at this stage either, of course). They'd be made after the Leeds game – a week after the Watford draw – but the booing crowd weren't aware of that. For them, recruiting in defence was a priority. Howe was in agreement, and spoke of his 'huge disappointment' about the result of the game:

> We'd played so well in the first half. We were energetic and we dominated the first half, playing with real threat. I really feel for the players. I think they were so desperate to win they went into a little

> bit of protection mode and we were in touching distance of a really important win but we didn't get it.

It was the same calm and thoughtful Howe that had been seen before and it was business as usual to focus on the next game ahead:

> We have to dust ourselves down very quickly, adjust our mindset and get ready for a massive game next week.

It was down to business, back to training and time to focus before the team travelled to Elland Road for their next game. And not only did they get a win, they got a glimmer of hope alongside their 1-0 victory against Leeds. After 75 minutes of opportunities for both sides, it was Jonjo Shelvey's 20-yard free kick that was enough to secure the victory. To hang on for a precious three points, to retain the lead was more than anyone could have hoped for, but they did, and the success sparked delight among the players and Howe as the final whistle blew. Trippier, again showing his appreciation to the travelling supporters, led the applause with Howe in front of their travelling fans. Afterwards, Howe was keen to remind those questioning their tactics, questioning his recruitment and questioning his style of management that this win represented a lot more than a few precious points:

> Today we learned that there's a resilience in the team. They're fighting for each other and fighting for the club. They have belief that we're not dead and buried and there's more to come. I'm so pleased for everybody connected with Newcastle that we won

> the game. It was a big match and hopefully it can transform our season.

Annoyingly, due to Norwich's win over Watford, Newcastle were still sitting in the bottom three, but with a training trip to Saudi Arabia coming up before they welcomed Everton to St James' Park at the beginning of February, this was a bright spark in a January gloom.

> Chris: For the first time in a long time, I enjoyed my Saturday evening. And Trippier and Wood were on top form. It was the start of things to come, babe.

Alan Shearer also spoke of the impact that Leeds game had, that 'jolt of optimism' it brought with it. Meanwhile, in hindsight, Howe too was able to reflect on it being a pivotal point in their journey:

> We really didn't know at the time how big that Leeds game was. Now I look back and go, 'Well, that was the turning point. That was the game that swung everything our way.' We won and, not only that, it was a real feeling of togetherness, because everyone contributed. It was a big day.

It was the start of several 'big days' to come. February proved to be the month of new beginnings. Playing at home to Everton was going to be a test of nerves, and despite going behind to a Jamaal Lascelles own goal, and after Jonjo Shelvey was fortunate to receive only a yellow card for a challenge on Anthony Gordon, Newcastle responded within 108 seconds through another own goal. It was the shortest gap between both teams netting an own goal in

Premier League history. But who cares about such statistics; the only thing that Newcastle fans around the country needed to be concerned about was that in the second half Ryan Fraser put Newcastle ahead in the 56th minute.

You could feel the roof being raised at St James' Park. Chants of 'Bruno, Bruno' also reverberated around the stadium as the fans clocked their other new signing on the bench. Having been named in the squad, the Brazilian international came out to the cheering crowd in the 90th minute. The applause and cheering and celebrations had only just died down as, ten minutes before, Trippier had scored an epic 25-yard free kick to the delight of the fans. A 3-1 win (and let's not forget, a consecutive win) had taken them out of the relegation zone at last. 'It's a big win,' grinned Howe. 'We're in a better place but we cannot get ahead of ourselves.'

It wasn't just the goalscoring that gave everyone hope, it was at last watching a team play that looked like they could be successful. They looked hungry for a win and they looked like that was an achievable goal, something their fans hadn't seen for a long while. A home win against Aston Villa five days later, thanks to another Trippier goal – another sweet free kick – allowed the fans another slice of celebration, and a reversal in their stats – they now hadn't lost a league game since Christmas. It wasn't a fairy tale ending to the match for Tripps, though, as the new captain sustained a broken bone in his foot (one that would see him out of action for eight weeks). But he'd gone out in a blaze of glory, and that win, alongside the draw against West Ham six days later, and then a further win against Brentford at the end of the month – a 2-0 victory, no less, with Joelinton and Willock goals in the first half – rounded off a pretty epic month.

Oh, and did we mention that Howe also won the Manager of the Month award? A well-deserved and well-timed achievement, the 16th time a Magpies manager had been given the accolade in Premier League history. Would the month of March herald such wonder too? Well, the first half didn't disappoint, as the first two games saw Newcastle earn themselves six more points. Fraser and Schär were the goalscorers against the Seagulls, within two minutes of each other, while the fans travelling to Southampton were in for a real treat when they witnessed Bruno's first full match. This was the rearranged match from the first game in January, if you remember, before Bruno had set foot in Tyneside, so the Saints would have faced a completely different team sheet – a sticky point for Ralph Hasenhüttl, whose team had now lost successive games for the first time since November. He argued that new signings should have been ineligible for this rearranged game.

But Covid rules were Covid rules, and this rescheduling meant that four of Newcastle's new players were now in the squad and Bruno was out for his first start. Southampton took the lead early on but Newcastle's travelling 3,300-strong support weren't worried. The chants and the cheers roared as Burn made some early challenges, then Chris Wood, seven minutes after the Southampton goal, responded with his first goal for the club to level the score by half-time. Rather than seem tired and try to hold on as they'd so often done in the past, Newcastle went on the attack. Jacob Murphy saw a shot deflected wide and, from the subsequent corner, Burn knocked the ball down into the six-yard box, where Bruno Guimarães, with his back to goal, effortlessly flicked the ball in with his right boot. There was absolute delirium among the away fans, who'd just witnessed a touch of class unseen for so long in the squad.

Bruno's goal saw the Toon win 2-1, their sixth success in seven matches, extending Eddie Howe's unbeaten streak to nine Premier League games and putting Newcastle ten points above the relegation zone. It was a moment of celebration but Howe was still clear that fans shouldn't get too excited just yet:

> We're not [safe]. Football changes very quickly, as we've seen for the positive. What we have done is put a gap between us and the bottom teams, but that's all it is.

However, there was a big smile when it came to discussing Bruno, who everyone very much liked talking about. He'd left the pitch with cramp after his wonder goal, to a standing ovation:

> I've not seen too much of that backheeling from close range. I thought it was a 'welcome to the Premier League' for Bruno because it was end to end, transitions and a very, very physical game. It will be a really good experience for him. He's a defensive midfielder, but a creative one. The reason we signed him was because we loved his way of playing, his eye for a pass and composure.

The final two matches of March didn't quite go to plan, but away games at Chelsea and Everton were both excruciatingly close defeats – both 1-0 and both in the last minutes of the game. Against Chelsea, the mighty Toon were only a few minutes away from securing a 0-0 draw against the then European and Club World Cup champions when, after an otherwise solid defence, Havertz scored in the 89th minute. Despite the late defeat, this was another sign of the progress Newcastle were making on the pitch and Howe was keen to stress that very point:

> It was really disappointing to lose our unbeaten run in that way, so late in the game as we'd been defending so diligently up until that point. It was a sucker punch at the end.

As Chelsea didn't have a shot on target for the first 75 minutes, Howe was also keen to stress that the performances he'd seen were impressive. He didn't want to dwell on the past:

> You have to just look at today, I was pleased with the performance. But in terms of what the players had given, I can't fault it.

More frustratingly perhaps was the loss against Everton on 17 March, again to a late goal, this one in the 99th minute of a game that ended up lasting 107 minutes due to eco protestors disrupting play. Howe later said:

> The second half is a big disappointment for us. We were off our usual rhythm. We've always looked to threaten in recent weeks but it didn't happen. The atmosphere was electric, the crowd kept with Everton, which was pivotal for them, I think. There were a lot of stoppages. We had the best of it in the first half and in the second half we didn't look or feel like the same team after what happened. It was a strange moment, never seen it before, we were out of sync. There has a been a lot of progress

> but we can't drop our standard in this league, it's so unforgiving.

During the game a protestor cable-tied himself to the goalpost. It certainly looked to have stopped the momentum for Newcastle, and to lose out in the dying moments was again a bitter pill to swallow. But for fans, remembering where they were at the beginning of the season, it put things in perspective. 'Things were never that bad,' confirmed Sam. 'But we wanted to keep going in the right direction. No one thought things would go tits up but we'd got used to losing in the last minutes of games before and we didn't want to do it again!'

An away hammering against Tottenham to start April was, thankfully, just a minor blip, albeit a 5-1 one. Fabian Schär had actually put the Toon ahead in the 39th minute but it seemed to wake up the sleeping Spurs, who responded with an equaliser four minutes later, then went ahead five minutes after that. Just six minutes later came another nail, then nine minutes later another. With seven minutes remaining the final nail was hammered home. But we don't want to dwell on the likes of those matches. There was the opportunity for some good results to come on their upcoming run of three home games, against Wolves, Leicester and Crystal Palace.

St James' Park knew they had a job to do over the next month and they were ready, vocal and raring to go. The team responded, thoroughly deserving their end to three straight defeats and denying Wolves any chance to touch the ball in the Newcastle penalty area in the first half. Then it was time for newbie Chris Wood to excite the crowd in the second half when he was awarded a penalty after being fouled by Wolves keeper Jose Sa. Wood slammed it home as the roars reverberated around the stadium and threatened to deafen the away team.

There could have been more celebrations, as Allan Saint-Maximin fired over the bar before Wood's goal and then Guimarães came close to adding a second. But it ended 1-0, a win that moved Newcastle ten points clear of the relegation zone – although celebrations couldn't begin just yet, as Burnley in 18th place had two games in hand. Howe told BBC Sport:

> It has put us in a stronger position but I still think we have work to do. The home games are key for us but we want to pick up points wherever we go. At this stage of the season it's about results. We're well aware we need to continue to get points. I think it's results over performances at the moment. There will be a time when we can evolve.

It was then a case of both performance and result at home to Leicester in the next game. The Foxes went ahead in the 19th minute, causing the home crowd to up the volume a notch and to focus on one of their favourite chants about one of their favourite new signings, Bruno. As the words 'Bruno's fucking magic, he wears a magic hat …' were heard around the ground, the Brazilian stepped up to show them how much he enjoyed their support, levelling the score on the half-hour. It felt like a long second half for everyone but in the fifth minute of stoppage time a low cross from substitute Joe Willock deflected kindly for Guimarães, who snatched the winner with an epic diving header. It was the first of that kind in his career, he said afterwards, and he was buzzing:

> What a feeling, what a game! To score two goals was brilliant. It was always my dream to play in the Premier League and I'm so happy for today. I want to be a legend here.

There was no doubting his legendary status among fans that day. The chants continued long after the whistle had blown and Bruno responded later in the year on X, which saw him wearing a straw hat, with the caption: 'Do you like my new magic hat?', followed by a laughing emoji. This was the sort of relationship that fans could get behind and they loved him. His impetus on the pitch and his love for the fans off it made him a firm favourite.

> Henry: He's such a talented footballer. But he does get a lot of bookings. I don't mind, though, Mum, I don't think people mind.

Henry's not wrong, Bruno did indeed get a booking for taking off his shirt in celebration of his header. But it was still a win and, not only that, five straight home victories, which meant Newcastle were on 37 points, now 12 clear of the relegation zone. Eddie Howe said about Bruno:

> Goals weren't necessarily one of the areas where we felt he would enhance us as a team, but he's scored some key goals for us. I'm really pleased with him today. I thought he was magnificent in every aspect, especially out of possession, because we struggled to get control of the ball for any large periods of the game. He's an incredibly passionate individual, he cares deeply whether we win or lose and I love that about him because you need

> players that wear their heart on their sleeve and are prepared to give you everything on the pitch. He's certainly one of those.

With one more home game in the month to go, would the Magpies make it three times a charm? Of course they would, and they'd do it in style, with Miggy Almirón scoring his first goal in over a year to secure a 1-0 victory, sending them up to 11th in the table. It meant they were all but guaranteed a place in the Premier League next season. Bruno Guimarães's lofted pass connected with Almirón in the 32nd minute, and he darted into the penalty area from the right before directing a sublime finish into the top corner. The stadium's reaction to the goal was testament to how much of a popular player Miggy has been, and Howe was thrilled for him:

> I'm so pleased, Miggy is an incredible professional. He had to wait for his chance and what a goal, the composure to finish was top level.

There were more chances for the home team, with Bruno and Allan Saint-Maximin testing Palace's Vicente Guaita in a one-sided first half. Joelinton excited the crowd early in the second half when he sent a header looping over the crossbar. Palace had emerged for the second half with greater urgency but a steady Newcastle defence kept them at bay. It was a point Howe was keen to make in the press conference after the game:

> We defended really well. For probably the last couple of months we've gone on an unbeaten run and our defensive resilience was excellent. We had a blip

> against Tottenham but after that we came back into some good defensive form.

The last time Newcastle registered six straight top-flight victories at St James' Park was during the 2003/04 campaign, Sir Bobby Robson's final full season in charge. But Howe didn't want to get ahead of himself:

> All we can do is win the next game in front of us. We've thrown everything at it and given it our all, and we want to do that until the end of the season. It's a great night for the football club and you can forget how hard it's been to get us into this position now. We have to look back with great satisfaction. You can very quickly forget where we were and where we've come from this season. It's been great to see the team move forward and develop.

Considering the position Newcastle were in when Howe took over in November – 19th in the table and five points from safety – reaching 40 points with five games to spare has to go down as a magnificent achievement. But Newcastle weren't going to digest that success just yet; they were still not quite in the clear and supporters could clearly remember what being in the relegation zone had felt like.

'We wanted to celebrate but we didn't want to … It was like waiting for a pub to open,' explained Craig rather succinctly while we were, ironically, sitting in our local. 'You get dropped off outside, you could see the staff getting ready and the pints being poured inside but you still had to wait a bit longer before the doors opened and you crossed the line. That's what it felt like. You couldn't quite relax until you had the first sip of that pint.'

That sip came when they travelled to Norwich three days later. Joelinton, in whom Howe had seen such promise when he first joined the club, decided to mark his 100th Premier League appearance in style with not one but two goals. Then the downing of the pint came when Bruno sealed victory with a third goal for the mighty Toon. It was Joelinton's third and fourth goals of the season and the away fans were delighted in his form. The opening goal came from a Saint-Maximin pass, which Joelinton placed into the top corner, and the second came from a tight angle just six minutes later, thanks to a Jacob Murphy ball. Howe was impressed, in his usual calm and unexcitable style (apparently the best thing about him according to my husband, as you don't want an overexcitable, dramatic manager):

> I have a great relationship with him [Joelinton]. He has so much ability and the two goals were great for him personally to score. He played dual roles and we love him to bits.

Bruno's goal came just after half-time when he chipped Tim Krul. It was a momentous moment for the team, the club and Toon Army fans up and down the country. The last time Newcastle met Norwich we came away with a 1-1 draw and remained bottom of the table. Then, we hadn't won in 14 games. Sports pundits had done their research and commentators across the networks were keen to reiterate the one important point of the season: no team had ever managed to stay up from that position.

So how had it happened? It was a question on everyone's lips. Howe had the answer:

> A lot of hard work, great team spirit, great unity and quality on the pitch as well. There are so many different factors but our supporters have played a massive part.

Indeed, the whole team knew that the away fans that day and the home crowd at matches at St James' were instrumental to results. It wasn't just that you could hear fans get behind you, but you could feel it. There's a sense of pure pride in the city and it's something Howe and his players felt as they finished the season in the clear. The supporters staying behind after the Norwich game after the final whistle to soak up their success was pretty unheard of then but something of the norm now. The players giving their shirts to supporters showed that they were aware of what the fans had done for them and that the success of the team was a combined effort.

For my father-in-law, the result meant he could start to relax.

> Grampy: We started winning. And then the Norwich game … it was enough. Once we knew we were safe, five or six matches to go, I could actually enjoy watching the games again. It was like I was watching with a different mindset. You weren't worried about people making mistakes. Personally, I think Dan Burn was a big part of that.

> Callum: Eddie Howe has flipped our club upside down and brought the best out in all the players. He'd bought players that some would think were a stupid idea, like Bruno, but who have done more for us that season than we ever asked.

For me, researching and spending hours going through interviews and chatting to fans about this moment, it's Howe that comes up time and time again as the one whose steering of the ship played a pivotal part. Yes, the money and the buying of the players was a massive thing, but those alone as credit oversimplifies what Howe did at that moment. Arriving at a club without a league win and with only six points from 12 matches, he began with five defeats in his first eight games in all competitions. And yet he was never flustered, he never floundered or blamed. He worked hard and continued to work hard. He proved that leadership is an action, not a position, and with four more games of the season to go, he wasn't finished.

Chapter 7

One for Sorrow, Two for Joy

'A magpie can be happy or sad: sometimes so happy that he sits on a high, high gum tree and rolls the sunrise around in his throat like beads of pink sunlight; and sometimes so sad that you would expect the tears to drip off his beak.'

Colin Thiele

ONLY LIVERPOOL and Man City boasted a better record in 2022 than Newcastle and it was those two teams that the Magpies had to face before matches against Arsenal and Burnley completed the season.

There was a buoyant mood at St James' Park as Liverpool were put under pressure by Newcastle from the word go, making the Reds nervous and the home crowd jubilant. It wasn't to last long, though, as a goal by Keïta in the 19th minute halted Newcastle's momentum, and although they came back strongly in the second half, it was to no avail. A 1-0 loss didn't seem that drastic against a strong Liverpool side, though, and the Toon Army's cheers and excitement during and after the game provided testimony to the pride they felt in a fight against one of the best sides in Europe.

It was a good opportunity for Newcastle to show what sort of threat they could pose to teams at the top of the table, although Howe was keen to stress that despite giving a good account of themselves, they could have done better:

> We weren't at our best but we competed well. We had a bit more energy in the second half and we were more aggressive and we knew that we needed to be stronger in the side areas. Improvement-wise, we were still in the game right to the end but we set our standards high and I'm slightly disappointed with general performance. What do I want from the final three games? I want a collective attitude – from staff to players. We have to show that we can compete for everything at every moment and we still want the points, we still want to climb in the league.

Knowing that Howe and the club were fuelled by high ambition for their last three games, it was a tough lesson that they learned on 8 May against Manchester City. In fact, it was a lesson City hammered home by outclassing Newcastle from the word go, although Chris Wood's early chance for Newcastle to take the lead may well have changed the dynamic of the game. However, a 19th-minute goal by Sterling started proceedings for City, one of two for the striker. Further goals from Laporte, Rodri and Foden followed in a 5-0 victory. For Newcastle, if there might have been one or two signs of promise, they'd quite simply been overrun by a team that seemed to be operating on another level. Of course, the travelling Toon Army were as ever in fine voice throughout, buoyed on by the return of Callum Wilson and Kieran Trippier from injury off the bench. It helped the mood ever so slightly.

> Chris: I was just happy seeing Tripps back. Forget about the score when we had him and Wilson come on you could see the impact they made. They're so important for us and the future.

But it's important to note that while the scoreline was perhaps a realistic reflection of the huge gap between the two clubs, and while there was clearly understandable optimism around Tyneside, it was peppered by the realism that there was no quick solution or smooth path to where Newcastle wanted to get to. They were on the right route, of course, but perhaps games like this showed how far in their journey they still had to travel. That said, relegation had been a very realistic prospect only a few months ago and now they were sitting in the middle of the table. There was a summer ahead of them to regroup and refocus, and with the prospect that anything was possible. Eddie wasn't despondent about the scoreline, which didn't really reflect his viewing of the game, knowing that they had 'good passages of play', but it was still a 'learning curve' for him and team:

> With the second and third goals … I was really disappointed from set plays, I think we'll kick ourselves. We know coming here Man City can hurt us in lots of different ways but we had a good spell when two subs came on, decent changes, good passages of play, tried to be positive in our approach, but the small details matter and they punished us. There was no better learning curve than playing

> Liverpool and Manchester City and they've taught us a lot about what we want to achieve. I don't think we're too negative about today; it's a learning of what areas we want to come back stronger and definitely grow in.

Sitting in 13th position in the table with two more games to go, a home match against the Gunners and an away fixture to Burnley, Newcastle were positive and fuelled with optimism.

'I remember not only enjoying the last few games knowing we were safe but actually excited about the new season already as I knew things were only going to get bigger and better,' recalled Ben. 'I was tempted to put on a bet that we'd win the league next season; it wasn't an outrageous bet, I would have got good odds!'

Arsenal were currently fourth in the table so Newcastle faced three of the top four teams in successive matches. There was therefore the prospect of another lesson for Newcastle to learn about where they stood among the giants of the league. Howe had only been in charge a matter of weeks when they faced the Gunners previously, but they were now a different side to the one that had lost 2-0 at the Emirates in November 2021. The focus on that game was all about survival; now the mindset was different and the players responded impressively to the question of whether they were up to competing this time, rather than enduring.

And compete they did, Howe revealing afterwards that it was 'one of the best performances since my arrival as manager'. It was Arsenal who went away defeated, having come to St James' Park hoping a victory would secure a place in the top four but realising that the Magpies were

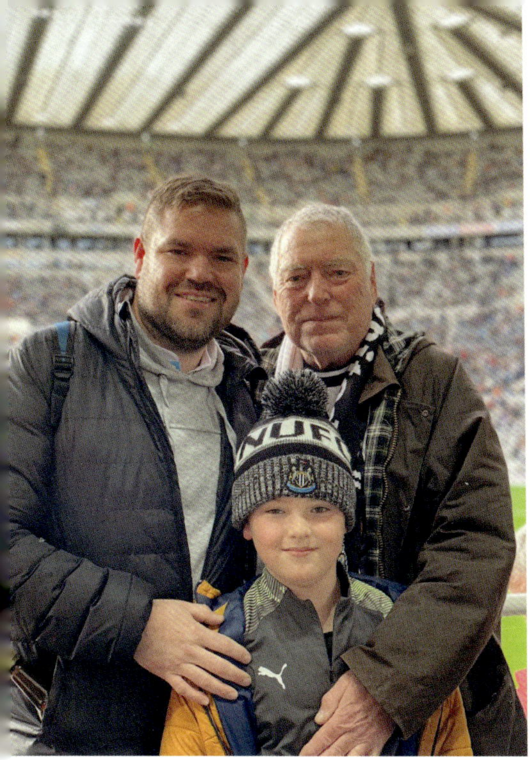

Three generations of Smiths at Henry's first Newcastle match at St James' Park in October 2021

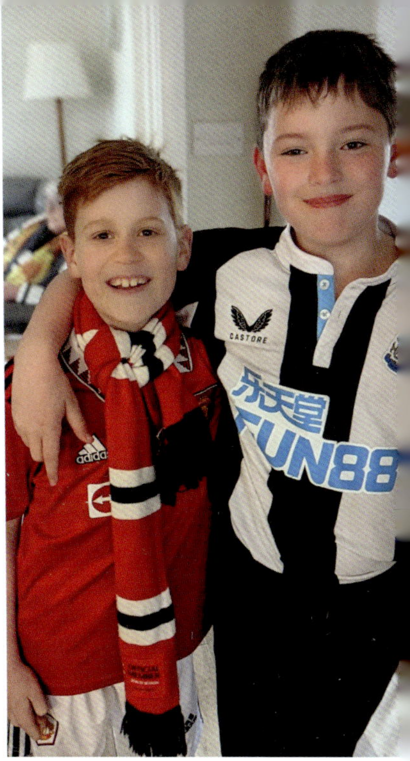

Best of friends Rory and Henry but rivals today! Manchester United versus Newcastle in the Carabao Cup Final, February 2023

Matchdays spent watching the game together, Grampy, Henry and Chris

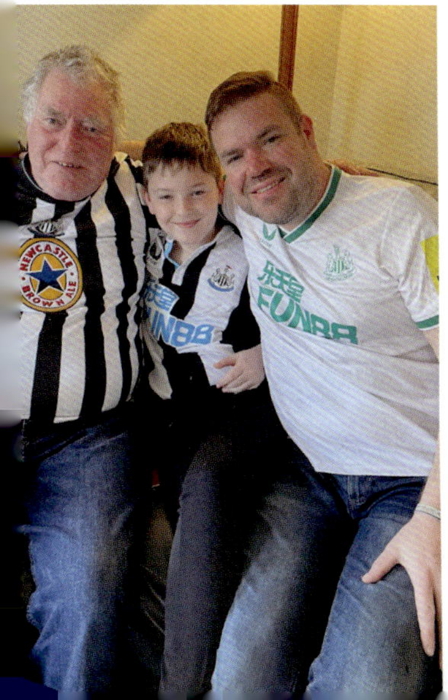

Chris and Henry watching the last home game of the 2023/24 season at St James' Park

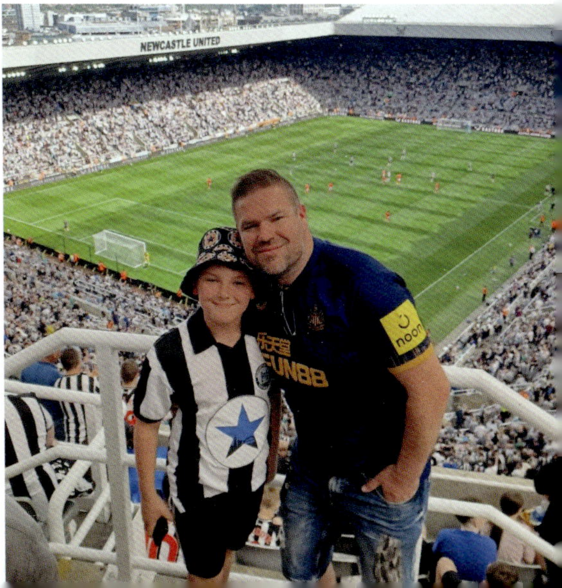

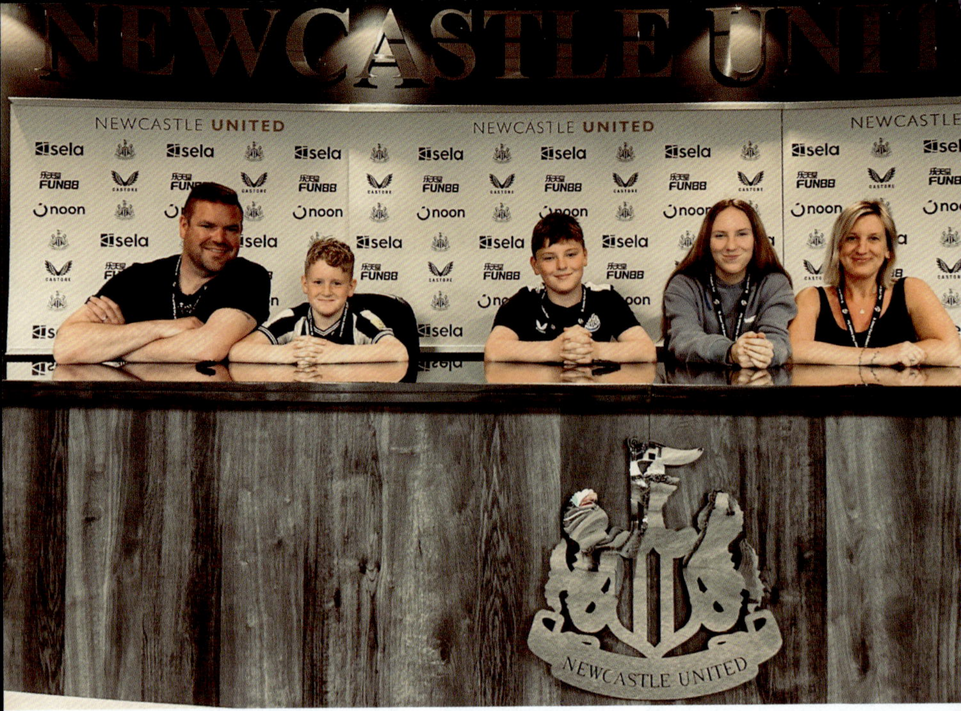

Family press conference behind the scenes at St James' Park

We are United

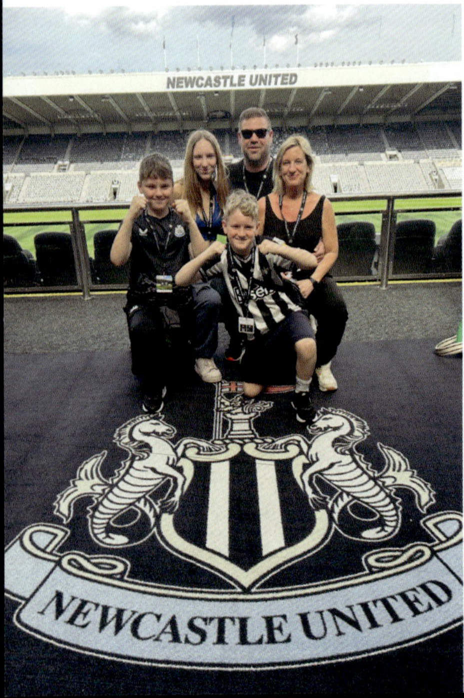

The tunnel out on to the hallowed turf, the steps stopping opposition getting the full force of the St James' Park crowd until it's too late

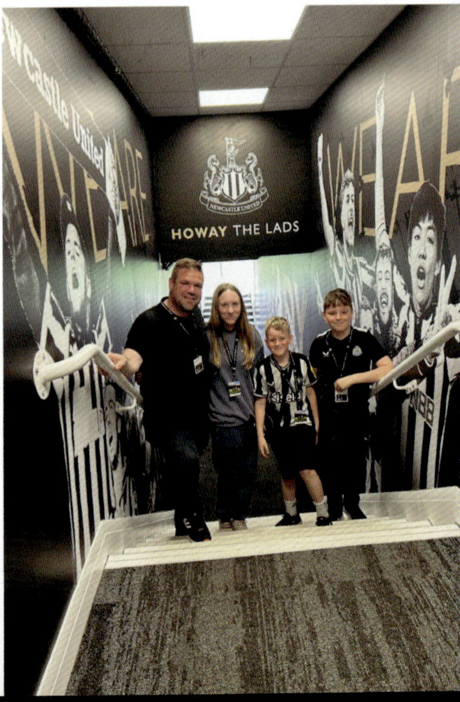

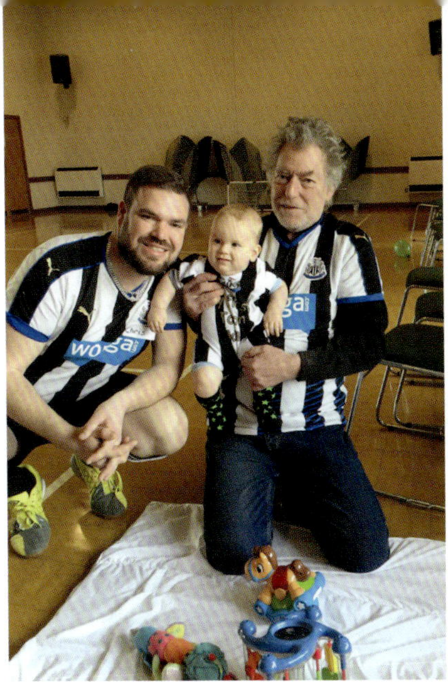

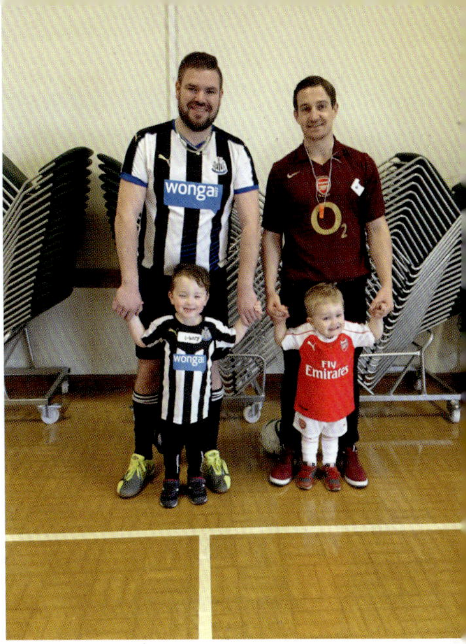
wonga
O2
Fly Emirates

Tommy, the youngest of the three to wear 'My First Toon Army' kit, 2016

Geordies and Gunners party… cousins and team-mates Henry and Albie 2016

Ashley who? Fans show how fed up they are with an owner who didn't invest, didn't care and didn't respect them, St James' Park, May 2015

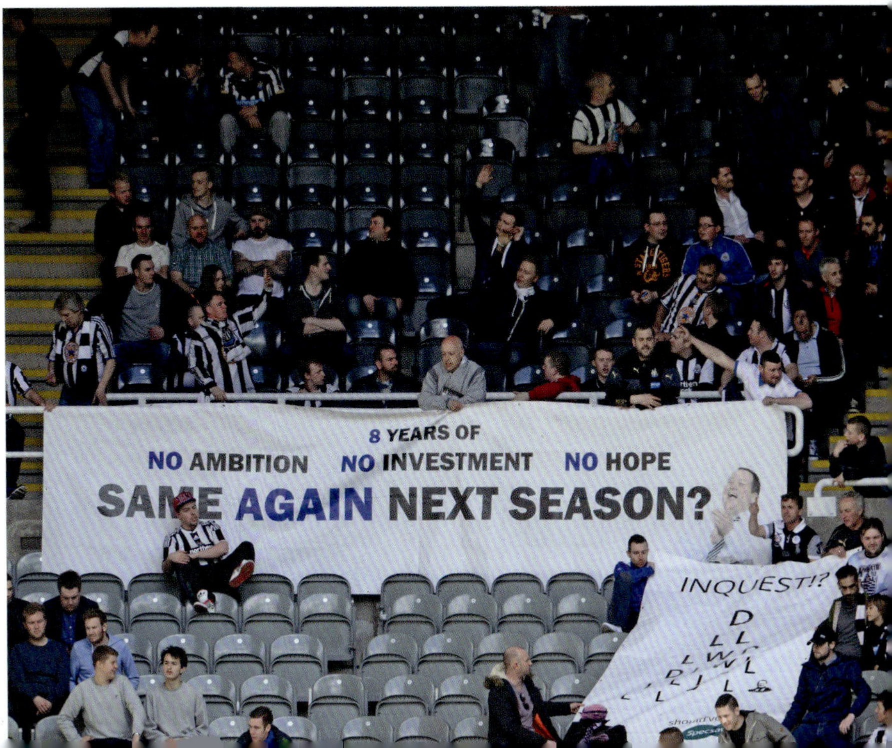
8 YEARS OF
NO AMBITION NO INVESTMENT NO HOPE
SAME AGAIN NEXT SEASON?
INQUEST!?

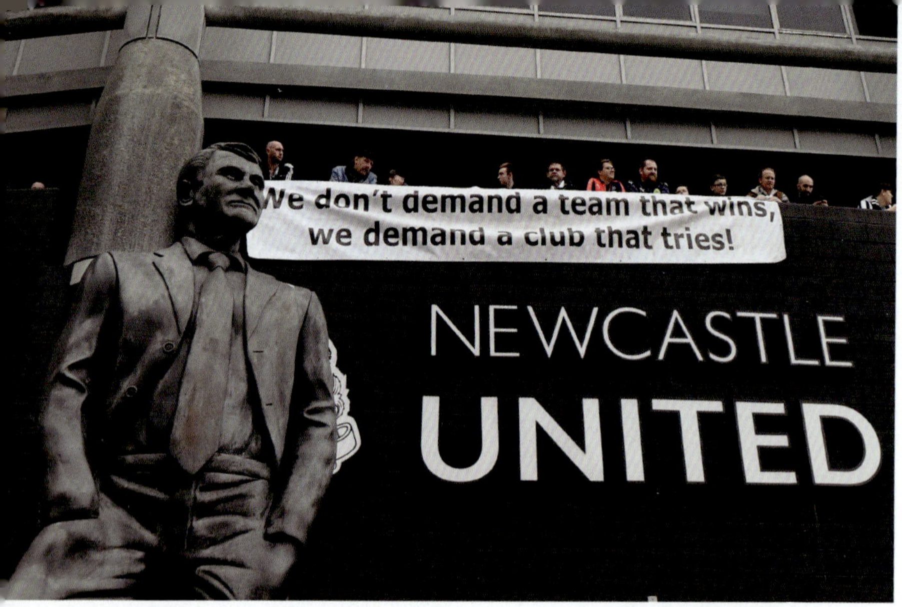
We don't demand a team that wins,
we demand a club that tries!
NEWCASTLE
UNITED

Newcastle fans expectant as a new era for the club beckons, October 2021

Thumbs up from the tracksuit manager, Eddie Howe makes sure the team know he is right there with them

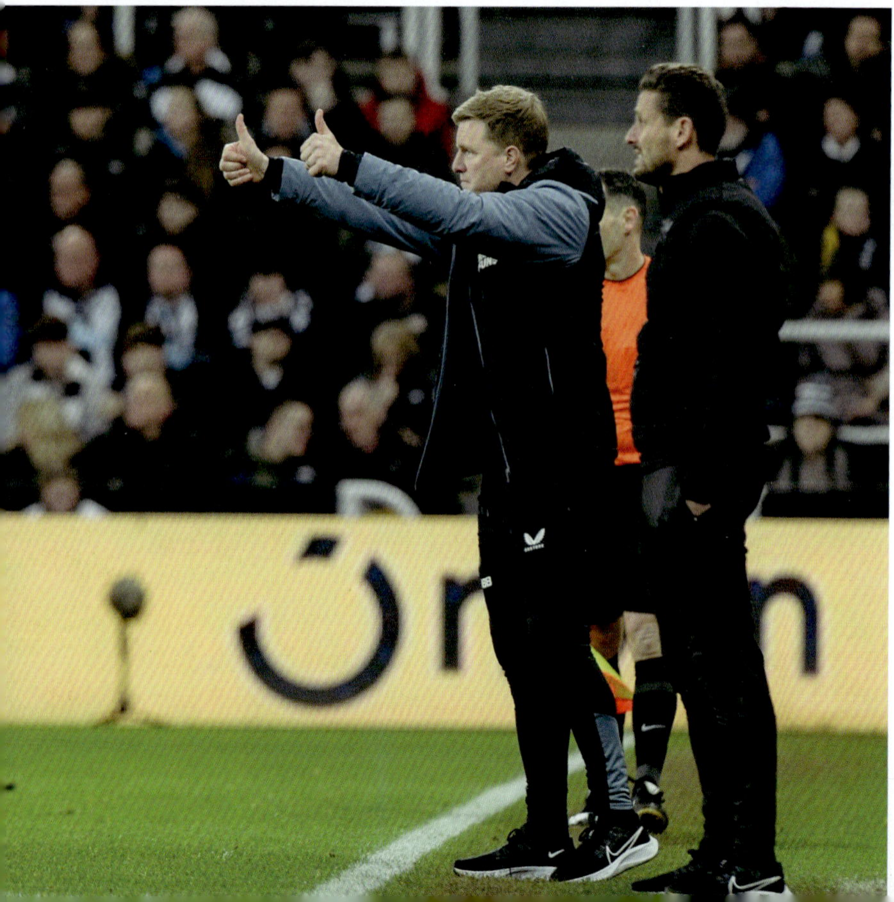

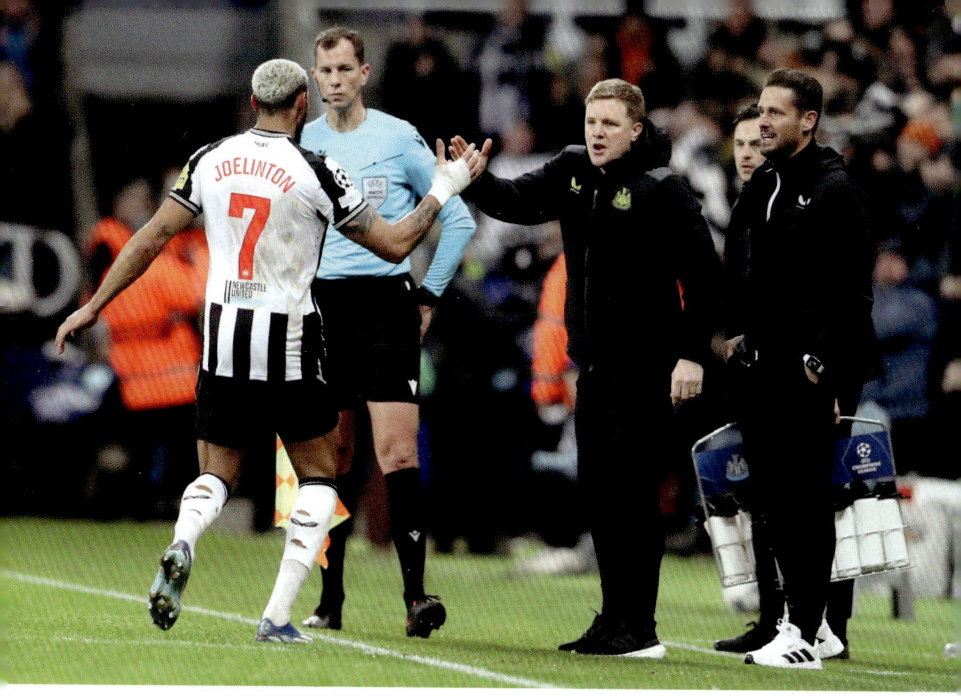

Joelinton celebrates with Eddie Howe after scoring the opening goal during the Champions League group F match against AC Milan at St James' Park

Newcastle United fans party in the street outside of St James' Park in May 2023 after Newcastle qualify for Champions League football

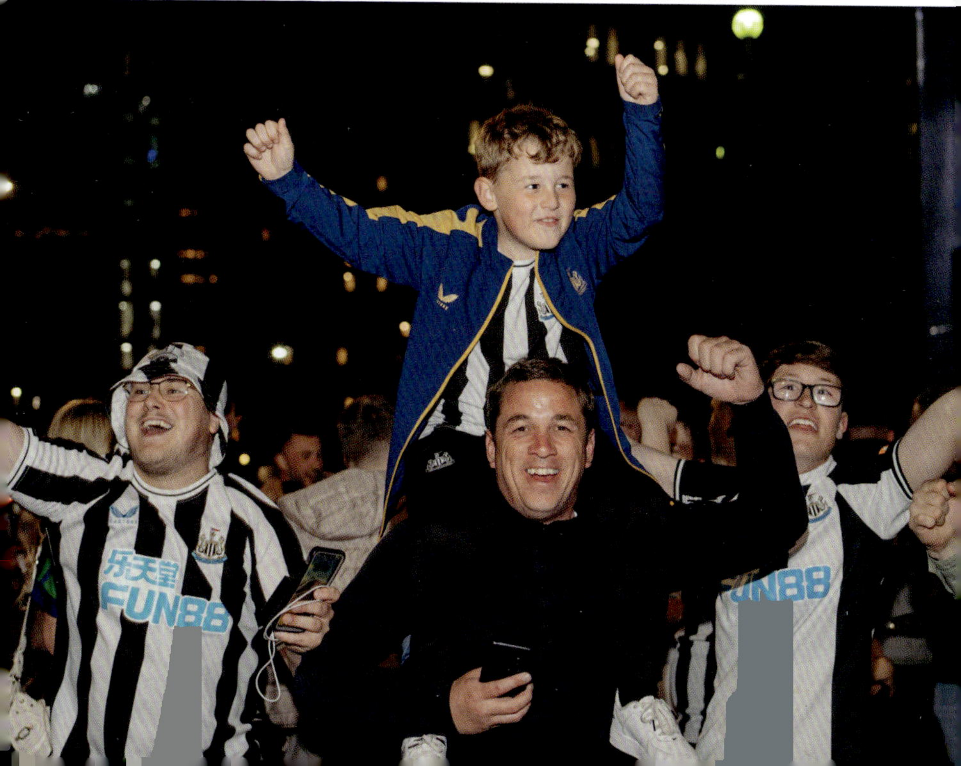

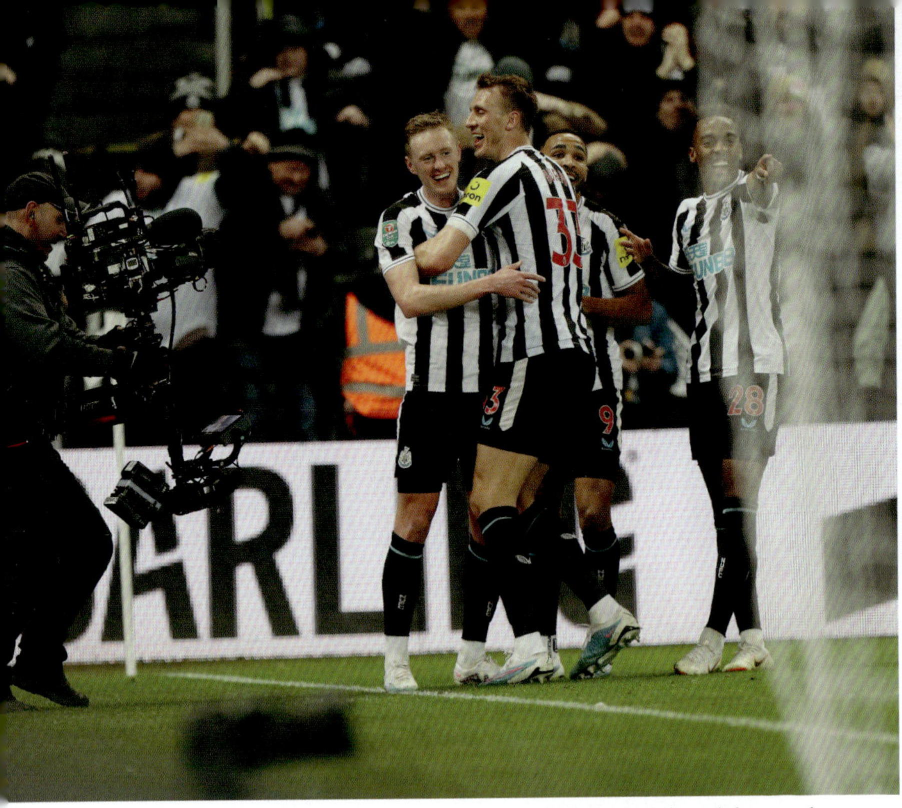

Sean Longstaff celebrates after scoring this and their second goal during the Carabao Cup semi-final, second leg match against Southampton at St James' Park in January 2023

The pied piper of Newcastle. Eddie has created a team ethos unmatched by any other club

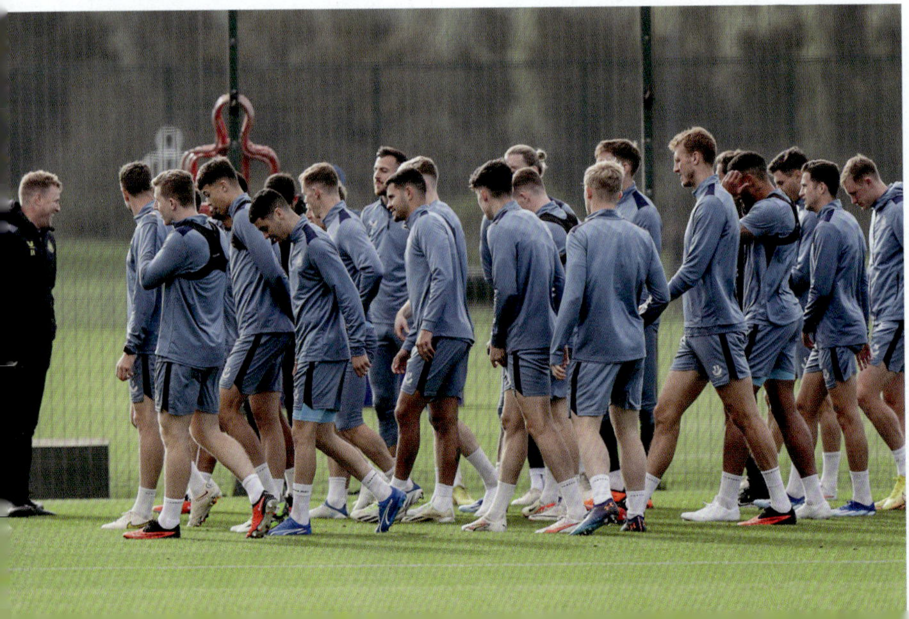

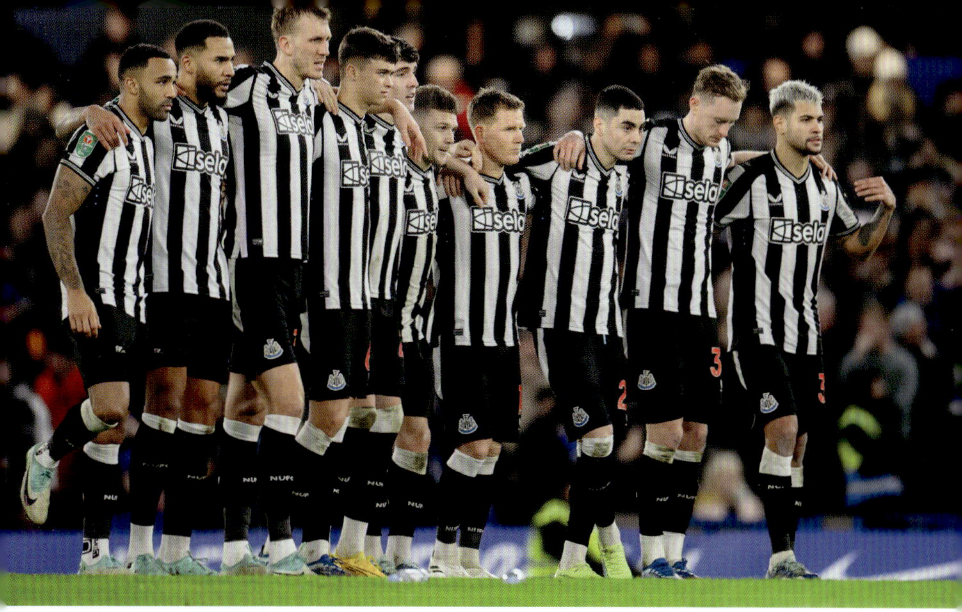

Chelsea v Newcastle United – Carabao Cup fifth round, December 2023 at Stamford Bridge. Players watch on during the penalty shoot-out against Chelsea

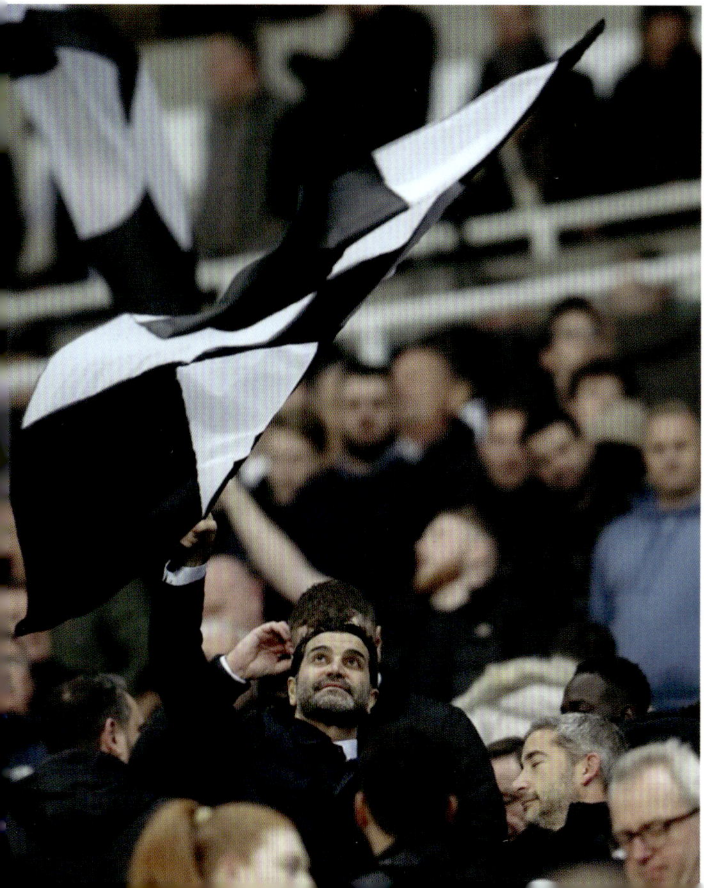

Newcastle chairperson Yasir Al-Rumayyan waves a 6ft flag and cheers Newcastle when they played Borussia Dortmund, October 2023

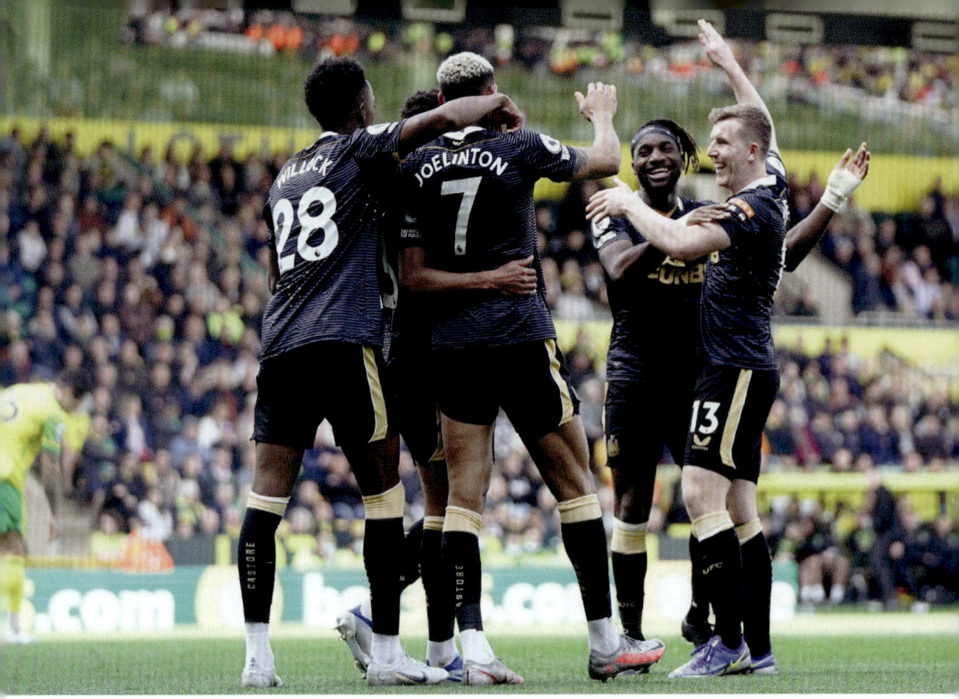

Joelinton celebrates with team-mates after scoring his side's second goal of the game at Carrow Road, Norwich, April 2022. The 3-0 win, the biggest of the 2021/22 season, saw them stay up in the Premier League under the guidance of Eddie Howe

Alexander Isak celebrates scoring his side's fourth goal of the game with team-mate Joe Willock during the Premier League match against Spurs which they won 6-1 on 23 April 2023

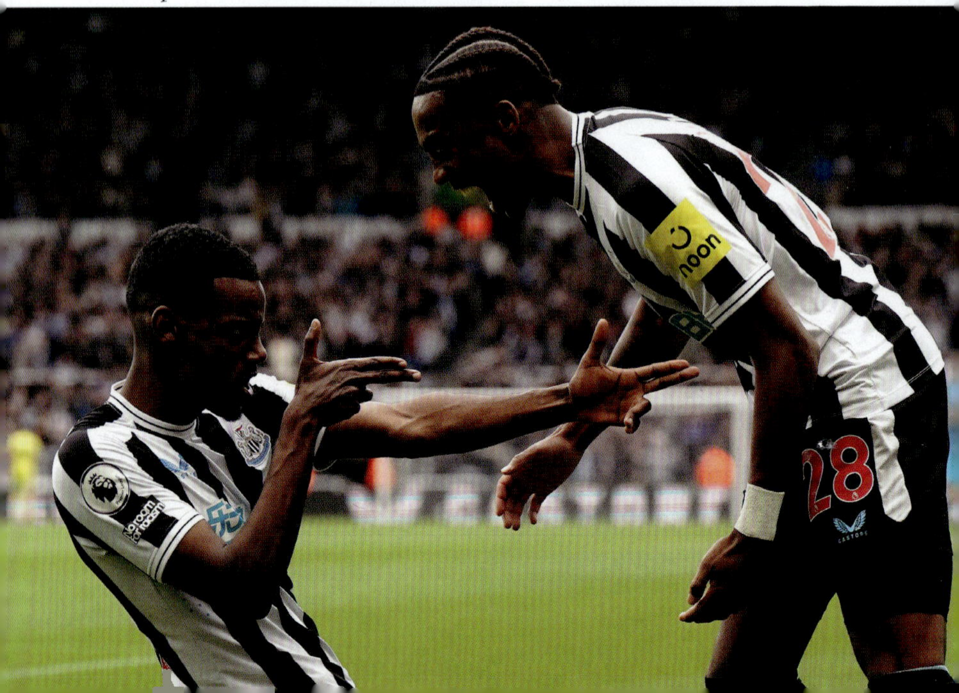

also on a mission – to give the home crowd a fantastic and positive lasting memory of the season.

In fact Arsenal were second best throughout the game and fell behind early in the second half when Ben White turned the ball into his own net under pressure from Callum Wilson, who was making his first start since 27 December. Bruno took the glory of the second goal when he drove into the net in the 85th minute, and Wilson also came close to capping a dream return from injury with a powerful long-range effort that went just wide. Arsenal didn't look threatening at all, and Martin Dúbravka was only tested once, by an Elneny shot in the second half. As one fan, Toby, pointed out in reflection, 'Newcastle seemed like they were enjoying themselves out there, it was great to watch. I wanted Wilson to score, coming back from injury – although he got bloody close!'

Howe was equally praising of the team afterwards, knowing full well that they'd proved something – to themselves, to their fans, to the owners and to the world – that they wouldn't have believed possible a few months ago:

> Full credit to the players. We were motivated by personal pride and we worked incredibly hard. It wasn't an easy game, Arsenal are a top-quality team. There were a whole host of things that have enabled us to turn the team around – unity, team spirit, togetherness are absolutely key. January helped us with the quality of players that came in but I would also say the mentality of the group played a big part too. They were determined not to get relegated and determined to achieve for everyone connected to the club. We've done that together.

It was the first time Newcastle had beaten a top-six side this season and Howe was aware of that significance:

> We knew that we hadn't achieved a result against one of the top six sides, that was something we hadn't achieved this season and in the future we will have to have the confidence to know that we can win anywhere. That will help us.

This being the last home game of the season, the biggest thanks went to the Toon Army, who had renamed themselves Eddie Howe's Toon Army. 'You give us hope on the pitch and we'll damn well give you a lot back from the stands,' said Tom. And Howe knew what difference that made. 'The minimum we can give them is 100 per cent effort every time we play,' he agreed when asked about the support the team felt from the fans. 'The challenge is to be consistent with that.'

'The team played like the crowd sounded,' confessed Alan Shearer in hindsight. 'It felt like a taste of what Newcastle could be.' It certainly gave those who were unsure of Howe a glimpse of a man who isn't a heart-on-sleeve wearer like Keegan and Sir Bobby Robson, but can still stir all the emotions that a football match can muster, as he said:

> I'm a very emotional person and I'm more emotional as I've got older, probably like we all do. If I put a film on … I'll cry straightaway over something like that. I think it's maybe when you have kids, you see life differently. But when it comes to football I'm able to control my emotions very well on matchdays because I'm always thinking about what my players need.

For part-owner Jamie Reuben, that last home game against Arsenal is also a day that will stick in his memory for a long time:

> The tremendous support we received after that match it was an amazing performance to cap off our season. It was a culmination of all our efforts – we had survived and succeeded. I went on to the pitch at the end and the atmosphere was truly amazing and it was a day I'll never forget.

In the final game of the season, the Magpies travelled to Burnley, who were hoping, in the dying embers of the campaign, to avoid relegation by keeping above Leeds on goal difference. But the mighty Toon, who, as Howe said after the game, knew all about final day results and reliance on other teams to win or lose ('we wanted to uphold the integrity of the league and it was important we played our part'), were on fighting form and secured a 2-1 victory to end their season in complete role reversal from how it started. Callum Wilson, named man of the match, scored twice – once with a calm penalty after Nathan Collins's needless handball, then from Allan Saint-Maximin's low, angled cross.

Burnley got a goal back when Cornet blasted in a volley – he'd already tried this before and been denied by Dúbravka – but one goal wasn't enough and Burnley's players hung their heads as Championship football next season became a reality, with Leeds winning their final match. At one stage it had looked likely to be Newcastle's reality too, of course, and that's what probably made this game all the more bittersweet – that Burnley and Newcastle had both been fighting to get out of the relegation zone from the beginning of the season and there was only room for one to succeed – the mighty Toon ended up 14 points above Burnley.

The only upset for Newcastle was an injury to Brazilian midfielder Joelinton, who was carried off the pitch on a stretcher after only ten minutes, although Howe assured fans that he'd seen the player, who was in 'good spirits' after the game.

And talking of good spirits, there was no denying the cacophony of emotions when the final whistle blew. It was probably a mixture of relief (after their early form), jubilance (they'd stayed up, they'd recorded some great results – in their last 18 matches it was 12 wins and one draw), combined with excitement (of what was to come).

'We finished on a positive note,' confirmed Howe in his last post-match interview of the season. 'We have very high standards, and we have a collective mentality and we approached the game in a very professional way.'

Not allowing Burnley to settle into the match was part of the game plan and it reinforced the idea that Howe was looking to be proactive, to play an attacking game and to not sit back and wait for the opposition to come to them. It was a line he'd said when he very first came to the club and it was reassuring that his stance hadn't changed – because imposing themselves in the game was something that Newcastle were doing very well.

Howe didn't want to get too complacent about the last game, as some parts he found 'quite scrappy', and the idea that there were always areas to work on showed how focused he was for the next season. But did Howe enjoy any time off in the summer? The question was put to him: 'Time off? I think it's important that I have some time to recharge my batteries but I had a year off and I'm relatively fresh and ready to go again.' And anyone reading between the lines might infer that Howe is someone who doesn't relax very easily, nor does he lose focus on his job at hand. The summer would be an interesting time for all involved with the club. The transfer market would play a big role but Howe was keen to stress that the squad had formed an incredible closeness with each other and there would need to be consideration about newcomers joining the club:

> We have an unbelievable spirit and mentality within the group at the moment and I definitely don't want to break that. My biggest challenge will be to harness and keep all the best bits of the second half of the season and to improve and evolve. I'm excited for the future. I think if we can be smart in the summer and try and keep the togetherness and the spirit that we've got, we can collectively improve. I think the future is very bright for the club. The main aim when I came in was to stay in the Premier League at all costs, and now I'm looking forward to next season.

Of course, ideas for who the club had their eyes on had long been discussed and planned for months – as far back as February when the league status of the team was still unclear. And now, as one season came to an end and another was only a few months away, it was all systems go for a newly energised, newly focused team.

'One day you will get your club back and it will be everything you wanted it to be,' Kevin Keegan famously said. And if you look back over the last few months, it certainly looked like this was the beginning of that hoped-for time. Gone were the downtrodden, disheartened fans, and in their place were ones who had pride in their team again, looked forward to a match, had hope and excitement for a new season, and who saw no reason that they couldn't now compete with the big teams – they had the money, they had the manager, they had the right owners.

Fans were now lauding the very players they put their hopes in on a matchday and felt that players had been reciprocating and enjoying the ride as much as the supporters. 'We'll be naming our children after these legends in the future,' confirmed Ted.

And talking of legendary, perhaps this is a good time to mention Wor Flags, who have dictated the atmosphere in St James' Park thanks to their epic flag displays that are jaw-dropping to everyone and anyone who can see them. They epitomise the emotion and enthusiasm of the crowd, deliberately trying to make displays that 'challenge, motivate and stimulate, both in terms of how much effort we put in but how it looks to supporters and the players'. It's probably no surprise that they or their excellent work (the orchestration of their displays are run like clockwork and are impressive to watch) help to both ramp up pre-match atmosphere or uplift and inspire the team – and intimidate the opposition.

> Henry: I saw loads just waiting for us to pick up and wave when we got to our seat, Mum. They were everywhere, you could just get one and be part of this massive group of people who were also waving the flags, it was great fun.

Wor Flags was created in 2017 when Gallowgate Flags merged with Wor Hyem 1892 (the singing section in St James' Park, Gallowgate's Block V) to create visual and audible support to the team. It's no wonder they boycotted the last year of Mike Ashley's ownership, pledging to stay away until the new owners came in.

The flags were certainly flying high as 2021/22 came to its conclusion, but now it was time to watch and wait. To see what – and who – was to come to the club in the new season.

Chapter 8

Summer Signings and Season Starters

'We do talk about Bruno …'

Henry

'THE CLUB means business again' was the mantra. It certainly felt like there was a new charge from the front as the summer months came into sight and so too the transfer window. There was a yearning about the club. The 'Geordie monster had been prodded' said many, and it was stirring. Having already spent a considerable amount of time sussing who they had their eyes on, the club was determined to hit the ground running when the trading period in the summer got underway.

There was already a strong team that Howe could focus on in the summer months before the new season kicked off, and he'd already voiced his summer holiday plans:

> We will remain very calm. We have to improve, we have to work incredibly hard over the summer to improve everything about the team to come back a stronger unit. The club has big ambitions but my job

> is to try and focus on how we do it, rather than just talk. And next season will be the proof.

So, on 1 July, after two weeks off but probably only half a day, if we know the man, Howe was keen to express his excitement over the upcoming new season after being back for the first day of training:

> It's good to be back. My voice is a bit croaky, but we had a good day back. Today was all about testing, like fitness, as we have our markers throughout the year, and tomorrow's second session about getting used to the ball again.

It was a typical, professional and down-to-earth summary by a manager who, when you recall Steve Bruce's haphazard attitude to training and gambling on player fitness, made everyone feel better about who was in charge. Points were what mattered only a few months ago when the club became close to careering into the Championship, but Howe oversaw a run of form that only Liverpool and Manchester City could better in the second half of the season. This was largely with the same group of players that his predecessor had failed to manage well enough – Joelinton being a prime example. He'd been mocked a mere matter of months before, but now he was like a colossus on the pitch thanks to Howe's vision in moving him into midfield.

Then there was the man who started the transformation, Kieran Trippier. No one was going to argue with the joy of welcoming a top England international into the fold. It started the revolution – for future investors and sponsors, players and, crucially, a new generation of fans. Tripps, however, put all the credit in Howe's direction, telling *Chronicle Live*:

> Eddie Howe has improved the club – that is there for everybody to see. What was important was that he got his first pre-season under his belt. He stamped his authority then on the way he wanted to play. Also the players he wanted to bring in. You can now see in the performances this season it really has shown.

And my husband had noticed one big difference:

> Chris: The amount of Bruno shirts I've seen around here reminds me of the amount of Beckham shirts that would be worn back in the day.

And we can definitely talk about Bruno (apologies if that's already been mentioned before – *Encanto* is a big hit in our house), who's a benchmark for what may be to come. And that was the big thing now, too; no longer was the club a stepping stone to the Premier League for overseas players, thanks to the people involved: the PIF, Reuben Brothers and Amanda Staveley. No longer was the stadium a laughing stock with the tacky signage of a shop linked to the name; even those not of a black-and-white persuasion would appreciate that. St James' Park was a far happier place to be. It wasn't just 'existing' as it had been previously, and, talking of happier, some new summer signings were bringing a big smile to the manager's face, as Howe confirmed:

> We've got three players who've come in, and I'm really pleased with new additions who'll strengthen our

> squad. They're the right characters for us. We want a minimum of two players in each position. I think competition brings out the best in everyone. Matt had a fantastic impact after joining on loan in January and made a big contribution to some excellent team performances. And Nick is an exceptional Premier League and international-level goalkeeper, so I'm very pleased to be adding strong competition to a very important position. There has been a lot of interest in him so I'd like to thank our owners and everyone behind the scenes for getting us ahead of the competition. I'm delighted he's joining us as we prepare for the exciting challenge ahead.

The first of the new signings was a familiar face in the shape of Matt Targett, the former Aston Villa left-back who'd been on loan at Newcastle in the second half of 2021/22. He was a key addition, having made 16 appearances, and Howe made sure they had a deal in place to sign the 26-year-old permanently for £15m. 'Having Matty on loan knowing they could keep him at the end of the deal was genius,' confirmed Luke. 'The club were thinking long term; it gave us confidence that they knew what they were doing, which was a feeling we hadn't had for a long time!'

Targett was equally pleased, having made himself a key member of the team. He felt right at home on the Tyne, as he confirmed on the club's website:

> I'm absolutely delighted to sign a four-year contract with this club. For me, it was an easy decision to make the loan permanent after the welcome I had from my fellow players, the staff, the supporters and the owners, so I'm really happy to be here.

It wasn't just Targett who was the, er, target. Newcastle were keen to strengthen their defence and made a big play for England goalkeeper Nick Pope – as did lots of other clubs in the summer – and finally managed to secure a deal that would see him play for the Magpies for the next four years. Pope had caught the eye as an experienced keeper who could cope under pressure. For the keeper, coming from recently relegated Burnley, it was a chance to remain in the Premier League.

> Tommy: Pope is the best in the business, Mum. He's my favourite goalie. And I mean, forever!

Meanwhile, Pope himself said:

> Now I'm here, I can't wait to get started. The deal has taken a couple of weeks to come to fruition but it got over the line really quickly, and I'm delighted to be here and I'm really looking forward to getting stuck into it.

With two June signings made, July brought with it another defensive rock to add to the squad in the shape of Lille central defender Sven Botman. He had been on Howe and the club's radar early on and was an integral part of the plan to strengthen the defence. They'd failed to secure the 6ft 4in player in the January transfer window, but with a fee of £32m, and a further £2.5m in add-ons, they finally had the final piece of the defensive jigsaw.

> Callum: I was excited about Botman. He came from a little club in France, he was young and he had lots of potential.

The Dutchman came on a five-year contract but negotiations with Lille had proved complicated and the Magpies had to beat off competition from AC Milan for his signature. Botman, however, knew Newcastle would be his new home and was delighted with the move:

> I can't wait to start this new adventure. This is the best day of my life, to sign a contract with Newcastle United. It's a day I've worked hard for and I'm very excited.
>
> Newcastle had a long-term plan to get to the top, for both me and for the club, and they play in the Premier League, which is the best league in Europe. The whole package is just perfect. I'm looking forward now to meeting the fans and also my new team-mates.

Eddie Howe confirmed:

> At 22, he already has solid experience at the top level but he's at a great age to grow with this team. I'm looking forward to getting to work with him and seeing him with his new team-mates.

It was a dream come true for all involved. 'Since he was a little boy, it was all about playing in the Premier League,' said Niels Botman, Sven's older brother. 'It was the opportunity to finally make his dream a reality.'

While the signing of three top-class players was a good start, it still felt like there was something missing. 'We were only opening the purse strings a little, it felt like,' said Lee. 'We were happy with the signings so far, of course, but they felt a bit modest with what we could be doing.'

Mehrdad Ghodoussi, in a tweet in June, simply stated: 'Patience is a virtue.'

The talk this season was to finish in the top ten … well, ideally in the top eight, especially as they'd been just seven points off seventh-placed West Ham at the end of the previous season. It wasn't unreasonable, it was a good solid aim, a focus and an idea that was tangible, even though Newcastle hadn't finished higher than tenth in the league since 2011/12, when they secured fifth place.

So there was definitely a feeling of 'something more' being needed to get from midway to the top half of the table. It what was later described as 'an increasingly fraught' search for reinforcements up front – Anthony Gordon and James Maddison proved beyond their reach, and Watford refused attempts to release Joao Pedro. But Howe was delivered the attacking signing he craved as his top striker target, Alexander Isak. The Magpies were deadly serious in their desire for the 22-year-old and completed a deal that saw a club-record fee of £63m to buy Isak from Real Sociedad. Tynesiders were elated.

> Chris: We were finally spending money and we were finally spending money on all the right players. It was like we were sending out a message to all the other teams and to all the other fans around the country: we're a serious team now, you have to take us seriously. It was a good feeling. [He was getting in his stride now.] We were all so weary of being thought of as weak; no, meek is a better word. Like we were only capable of being played against, of sitting back and taking a hammering. No one thought we were a team that could put up a real fight for a long time. But now we weren't lacking anymore, it was like a

> sleeping giant had been awoken and the club was being 'seen' for the first time.

I've got to say, it was quite a speech from Mr Smith. He had been to the pub, however.

The serious nature of the club is a good point to expand on, although at the time of writing this I think the focus should be on the way the club seems to be now setting a precedent in the footballing world. It's not just serious, it's yearning and it's fiery and it's vibrant. The owners seem to be pioneers when it comes to visionary tactics on how clubs are owned and run. Amanda Staveley, for example, spoke at the Bloomberg Power Players Summit in Saudi Arabia in March 2024 and addressed FFP regulations within the Premier League and how they're impacting Newcastle's growth since the takeover. Staveley was adamant that a revamp was needed:

> It's a difficult time because there's just been so much focus on sustainability that people have actually forgotten that we're providing entertainment and we've got to grow this business. Sometimes, when you over-regulate, you can slow growth and I think we have to make sure that we get the right balance between the right regulatory environment, the right rules and the right Financial Fair Play rules that promote growth. That's the only way you're going to get great football.

Touching on investing in football clubs, namely those that belong to the English top flight, she acknowledged that Premier League clubs 'are very much seen as financial assets'. You just have to look at the powers that rule Newcastle to get a fancy glimpse into that reasoning.

She also added that the 'regulatory environment [the one created by FFP rules and constraints] has allowed private equity to come in and invest'.

If the PIF were to invest in another club playing in Europe, they might encounter problems in having both clubs under their umbrella competing in the same tournament, such as the Champions League, but Staveley recognised that it would help Newcastle in 'getting players through our academy system' and a multi-club model would 'be very helpful in terms of allowing us to buy and have players as part of our journey earlier on'.

Staveley also expressed interest in the idea of investing in a Saudi Pro League club in addition to a European one, perhaps taking advantage of the already established relationship with the PIF at Newcastle. Who knows what the future might hold? But perhaps it's safer for now to go back to where we were, Isak joining as the new 2022/23 season came into view.

Howe was desperate for his new striker to be given clearance for selection in the game against Liverpool, their fifth fixture of the season, telling reporters:

> It'd be great to see him involved. We're in the hands of other people so we hope it gets done before the game. The cut-off is 75 minutes before kick-off so it could go down to the wire. We've had minimal training with him between games but what he has done he's done very well. He's looked bright, keen and shown us little flashes because the sessions have been quite light. We're certainly excited by him.

The excitement had built from the training camp in the summer. Howe was keen to get the team focused, with several pre-season games, which allowed for the training facilities to be worked on:

> Pre-season friendlies, these games are really important. We want to see the team play and develop and focus on how we want to play the game. The schedule is based around our training ground, which is having work done.

Having work done wasn't, in this case, a euphemism. It was actually happening. It's telling that the new owners saw the club's base in Benton and agreed it wasn't fit for purpose. This wasn't something we hadn't heard before. There had been plenty of false promises from various Mike Ashley stooges down the years that they wanted to improve the academy and training ground, but to no avail. Quelle surprise. Rafa Benítez came out with the damning line about the false promises: 'After three years they painted the walls.' But the new owners have made good their word. As they have done in bringing the women's side to the forefront, in celebration of their achievements. It was the new owners who welcomed the women's team on to centre stage, to showcase them at St James' Park and to promote and recognise their ever-growing list of achievements. It's been hardly mentioned in the national press but is widely talked about among the Toon Army contingency. The PIF, and Staveley in particular, stayed true to their word, promoting each win and accolade on social media with the gravitas it deserved. And it should definitely be a book in its own right.

* * *

> We want the fitness of the players to be sufficient for the league that we're in. Tactically, we want to be

> ready to play the game in the way we want to play. That means lots of hard work behind the scenes to make sure the team is ready to perform at its best.

Howe had set the intention of the team at the beginning of July. And now, with the new signings in place, the hard work had to begin.

Before they embarked on two home pre-season friendly fixtures ahead of the start of the 2022/23 Premier League season – a double-header at St James' Park against Atalanta on 29 July, before playing Spanish side Athletic Bilbao the following day – they'd enjoyed some more pre-season matches against local neighbours Gateshead FC. Winning 5-1, it was a good opportunity for Howe – who fielded two teams over 90 minutes – to put into practice some of the plans he'd established for the season. They didn't have their three new arrivals but the trio were going to be part of the pre-season camp in Austria as they looked to ramp up proceedings for another match, against 1860 Munich at the picturesque Saalfelden Arena Bürgerau, before facing Mainz (which, incidentally, didn't go so well, the Magpies losing 1-0).

Then it was time for a training session in Portugal with Burnley at the Portuguese Football Federation's Cidade do Futebol, the positive momentum from the end of last season continuing into the current pre-season campaign. Everyone was in good spirits. They took on Portuguese giants Benfica at the famous Estádio da Luz, winning 3-2, before heading home towards the end of the month to play those two home friendlies in two days against Atalanta and Athletic Bilbao.

The Magpies and Atalanta had both finished eighth in their respective domestic leagues the previous season, with Atalanta also reaching the last eight of the UEFA Europa League after being eliminated from the Champions League during the group stage. Known formally as Athletic Club, Basque-based Bilbao also came close to cup success during the 2021/22 campaign but lost to Real Madrid in the Supercopa de España Final, having lifted the trophy the previous season.

Both friendlies were a big success for Newcastle, and playing at home with large crowds (40,000 for a pre-season!) the team had a boost for the season to come, as a delighted Eddie Howe exclaimed:

> Huge respect for everyone for coming and supporting us in the numbers that they did. It's a brilliant thing for us. Hopefully we can show them that the work we have done pre-season will mean that we're ready for next week.

The next week, of course, being the start of the new season, which kicked off earlier than normal, on 6 August, due to a mid-season World Cup in Qatar. It was all systems go and Tynesiders were ready …

Chapter 9

Gimme, Gimme, Gimme a Striker from Sweden

'He's got a bit of the X factor about him.'

Eddie Cowell (sorry)

THE BUILD-UP to the start of the new season was exciting enough, but throw in the last-minute signing of Alexander Isak and the tempo was rising. Howe, rarely given to hype, was keen to express his excitement over the new signing:

> He looks like a special player. He has pace, technical ability, dribbling ability. I think he's capable of scoring goals. He's technically very good and has a mix of qualities I really like in a forward player. For such a young player, he's had a lot of experiences thrown at him, playing for big clubs in Germany [Borussia Dortmund], the Netherlands [Willem II] and Spain [Real Sociedad]. The English game will suit his profile. He's a really good athlete with a host of things going for him and his best years are ahead of him. He's a very exciting signing for us.

Howe was keen to see his new wonder striker make his debut against Wolves, which was to be Newcastle's fourth fixture of the season, on 28 August. But we're getting a bit ahead of ourselves. Let's head back to the beginning of the month and the start of the season was off to a flyer when the Magpies welcomed to St James' Park newly promoted Nottingham Forest, who were back in the Premier League after 23 years. It was quite a return for the club, facing a Toon side that were out and raring to go on home turf and who pummelled the opposition 2-0 (let's face it, it could have easily been five or six the way Newcastle came out firing on all cylinders). It was a great start to the season, only their second opening-day win in ten attempts, but the following game against Brighton was slightly more flat and ended 0-0.

There was, however, then an almighty 3-3 draw against Manchester City on 21 August, which cemented the idea that Newcastle were here to compete, not just exist, but compete. Going one down early on wasn't the best start but boy did the crowd filter on to the pitch and bring the game back. On the pitch it was mainly thanks to Saint-Maximin, who assisted in the next three goals, as Newcastle went ahead 3-1, with goals from Almirón, Wilson and Tripps. It was yet more evidence of the sleeping giant having been awoken. Although City came back to take a point, Howe was happy after the match:

> We scored some great goals. I was absolutely delighted with the effort and commitment, everything the players gave. I'm sure for the neutral it was an incredible game. For us as managers you're torn because we were 3-1 up and you're desperate to win, but we needed something from the game and I think the players deserved that.

New goalie Pope had a massive game too, and former Magpies goalkeeper Shay Given was full of praise for the player:

> He strikes me as someone who doesn't do anything flash. Even in the last minute, he comes and claims the cross when City were pushing hard, to take the pressure off. He brings that calmness, nothing fancy, but he made some big saves today. He's 30 years of age, there's still plenty of room for improvement and I think Eddie and his staff will be working on that.

The press were keen to point out that Howe had spent in excess of £200m since succeeding Steve Bruce less than a year ago but equally praised the fact that he was adding players to positions that would mean there was always a contingency plan and they wouldn't be left short in any particular area. Isak and Callum Wilson, for example, could prove different enough in their style of play to eventually play together. Wilson, unfortunately being injury-prone, was struggling in the Man City game with hamstring issues, as Howe explained:

> Callum was feeling his hamstring at half-time. Just a tightness, nothing more than that, but we were aware looking at him second half he wasn't fully opening up. We felt at that moment the team probably needed someone who could fully sprint. We wanted to protect him from serious injury. I back Callum 100 per cent, I've known him for a long, long time and have never met anyone with a better attitude or a better professional. Callum's such an important part of our future.

Being without his principal striker, if only for a few games, you could see why Howe was keen to bring Isak on for his debut in the next league game against Wolves, but the transfer paperwork was the hold-up. Newcastle had submitted Isak's registration to the Premier League before the Friday 12pm cut-off point; however, the decision on whether or not he could feature was subject to a work permit and international clearance – and it didn't come in time. Although Isak did travel with the team to Molineux, it was frustrating for the newbie, who was keen to get on with the job he was desperate to do. 'Obviously it's a bit frustrating to travel with the team, not knowing if you can play,' he told *The Athletic*. 'I prepared as if I could play, but you can understand it's not the same.'

The Wolves game, which ended in a frustrating 1-1 draw, also drew attention as it was the first time the team had played in this season's green-and-white third kit. While many maintained that the takeover was more about the end of the Ashley era than who came in, the press were still keen to draw the connection with the club and Saudi Arabia – especially as the third kit had a great resemblance to the Saudi Arabia national team kit. Amnesty International said that by wearing it there was 'clear evidence' of 'sportswashing' by the Saudi state. Others didn't agree.

> Steve: I saw the photos of the kit when they were leaked earlier in the year on social media. I didn't have a problem with it. We've played in many away colours over the years, it's nothing new.

And the ever-diplomatic Howe didn't rise to any stirred-up press stories either:

> I'm aware of the criticisms. I think from my perspective it's not something I've had any control over. We were very aware when we went to Saudi Arabia that the interest in Newcastle is huge. I know I'm making an assumption here but our kit manufacturers have probably acknowledged that, and hence why we've ended up where we are.

Meanwhile, what was coming close to a five-day wait for Isak's clearance to play – not helped that it was over a Bank Holiday – ended on Wednesday lunchtime, around seven hours before kick-off against Liverpool. Isak's work permit had been granted. 'It was a nice disruption,' Howe admitted. 'We were waiting yesterday and today and with the silence fearing the worst.'

Isak had trained as a centre-forward during team-shaping sessions, regardless of whether confirmation of clearance was received, and in the end Newcastle waited until 75 minutes before the match to name him in the squad as they handed in their official team sheet.

'I was well happy to see him on the list,' remembers Dan. 'I heard he had a dead powerful strike on him. We needed him too, with Wilson and Bruno off.'

As debut matches go, this one would probably be up there as one of the finest. The result didn't go the way Newcastle wanted, losing 2-1 to an added-time goal, but such is the cruelty of the game. This was all about Isak's introduction to the black-and-white gang and he was that fluid that he looked like he'd been playing alongside his team-mates for years. And scoring for your new team on your debut match after just 37 minutes? Well, it was a moment that bridged that gap from rest to the best in jaw-dropping fashion. Isak's strike of unerring accuracy and considerable power came from a Longstaff through ball and hit the back of the net in a fashion of which Alan Shearer would have been proud. Away supporters believed they might witness an Anfield victory for the first time in years when he scored again but the goal was questionably deemed offside. After that, Roberto Firmino scored past Pope to level the scores. It looked as though it was going to be a draw, but Liverpool somehow scrambled a goal in the eighth minute of added time from late substitute Fabio Carvalho. It was a cruel finish for the Magpies.

'Liverpool were very, very lucky. Newcastle didn't deserve to lose that in the 98th minute' came the response from most of the pundits.

But Isak, who was disappointed not to have had his 'dream debut', as he later told reporters, was warmly welcomed by the travelling Toon Army before, during and after the game. The Sweden flags were flying in his honour and the chant had been prepared. To the tune of ABBA's 'Gimme, Gimme, Gimme', the words: 'Gimme, gimme, gimme a striker from Sweden. He's our number 14 and he plays in attack. Gimme, gimme, gimme a striker from Sweden. First name's Alexander and his surname's Isak' rang around Anfield after his goal.

And it has been sung with gusto ever since. Isak showed his gratitude to the welcome before the match began. After taking part in a warm-upand receiving whisperings of encouragement from Graeme Jones, the assistant head coach, Isak and his fellow attackers practised shooting. Simon Weatherstone, the first-team coach, laid the ball off to the forwards, who took a touch and shot at either Karl Darlow or Mark Gillespie, and Isak was looking good. But before returning to the changing rooms with the rest of the team, he ran to the cheering fans in the away end, clapping his hands over his head in appreciation of their cheers and waves. Those cheers continued as he and the team later came out on to the pitch for his debut. And he couldn't have asked for a better start.

By scoring the opener during the galling 2-1 defeat, Isak joined a prestigious group of Newcastle United strikers who have found the back of the net on their Premier League debut, including his team-mate Wilson, who scored against West Ham in 2020.

> Henry: The first goal he scored, in his first match, I was like, 'Dad, he's going to be a good player.' And then he scored again but apparently it was offside.
>
> Chris: Newcastle deserved more from that.

If you took away the small matter of the scoreline, it was encouraging. Isak was encouraging. What he achieved without much training and without some of his talented team-mates was encouraging. Howe was also impressed:

> I wasn't surprised. I know what he's capable of. He looked a threat and his pace was a key outlet for us. He gave us that pace in behind that teams need.

But the scoreline? That was hard to forget. Even for the most fluster-free manager, losing 2-1 in the 98th minute was a kicker. And how do you, as a manager, put your frustrations to one side when in the 98th minute you lose 2-1? It was a rhetorical question but one that Alan Shearer managed to get the answer to:

> That's not one of my strengths. After the Liverpool game, the ending lived with me. It's still probably with me now. And it may be one of those moments that you never truly move on from. I was replaying the last couple of minutes, thinking, *What could we have done differently?*

It wouldn't be the last time Howe would be frustrated by results sitting in stark contrast to how the team had played. The following week when Crystal Palace visited St James' Park, Newcastle were on the wrong end of a terrible VAR call that left them with a bitter 0-0 draw. It's not a new thing to moan about the VAR system; it's an infuriating system that you love if it helps your team but, bloody hell, you won't hear the end of it if it doesn't. It's a system that's meant to iron out mistakes but, actually, is still very vulnerable to human error. After the Crystal Palace game, Howe was equally unimpressed by the workings:

> The problem is that they're missing the big decisions, the clear ones like that affecting games, and then getting involved in ones they shouldn't. It's become a mess.

The 'mess' from that VAR call meant that Newcastle were sitting in 11th place in the table. In context, of course, this was a far better position than where they'd been the previous season but wasn't an accurate assessment of their performances so far.

So, it was perhaps bittersweet that it was a VAR decision that awarded Newcastle a penalty when they hosted Bournemouth in September to give them a chance to level the score in what was a frustratingly lacklustre game. Newcastle created lots of chances – Trippier shaved the outside post, Joelinton went closer and Ryan Fraser even closer, but to no avail. When the Cherries scored early in the second half the home crowd were roaring in upset because they knew what the players knew: they deserved more. They were treated to Isak taking the penalty, which gave them hope and a chance to chant for their newbie wonder signing, but there was a fair amount of booing as the final whistle blew. It was their fifth stalemate from seven league games and Howe was sure of one thing the team were lacking. 'We didn't have that zip feel about us that we have done at times this season,' he said afterwards. And it was true, something wasn't quite clicking.

Perhaps October would be different. With the World Cup looming there was the opportunity to achieve some good results before the break and to get back a bit of control and momentum. That came on the first of the month in what was then a clear indication that the team had been working hard on finding that zip, and had found it at Craven Cottage against Fulham. Callum Wilson, back from injury, and Longstaff both banged in goals that gave the away fans something to cheer about. But it was Almirón who held the 'magic' of the game with two goals that saw the Magpies win 4-1, jump up the table to sixth and, a week before the anniversary of the takeover, gain their second win of the season. Howe told BBC Sport:

> It's been a very difficult two weeks. But it didn't show in our performance. Right from the start we had a good feeling, with good energy, and created chances early on. I'm delighted for Miggy, he's such an infectious character. His work sort of epitomises

> our play, so it was great to see and he's capable of doing magical things.

And the magic continued. The day after the Tynesiders enjoyed the anniversary of the takeover, they had a home game against Brentford and went one better than they had the week before, beating the Bees 5-1. Bruno started the goal haul after 21 minutes before Murphy added to the tally seven minutes later. While the visitors tried to put up a somewhat lacklustre fightback in the second half, it was quickly snuffed out by another Bruno strike 11 minutes into the half before a late Almirón goal and a Pinnock own goal secured an epic victory. Bruno chants rang out as the knowledgeable home crowd knew what an instrumental part he'd played today as well as the success he'd brought the team on the pitch since joining the club. The stats spoke for themselves: since his Premier League debut in February, no Magpies player had scored more than his seven goals, and that from midfield. 'He's top quality in every aspect – his personality, his performances on the pitch,' said Howe. 'I thought he was outstanding today.'

While his two goals stole the show and the majority of the cheers, it would be unfair not to mention his ability to lead from the front, with and without the ball. Apart from Botman – who was finally making a spot in Newcastle's defence his own – no player on either side had won possession on more occasions or won more duels than Bruno, so often described as the beating heart of Howe's side.

'He's bloody outstanding,' said Danny. 'Just brilliant. He gets the team behind him.'

The dynamic among the team had been spotted by fans following Howe's arrival – there was no one leader in the team on the pitch or in the dressing room, but there was a leadership group among the squad, which meant a shared ownership of responsibility. And you didn't have to be playing to lead the team, it wasn't just on one person's shoulders but more a collective effort.

'Bruno is my favourite player,' joked Sean Longstaff, when asked by schoolchildren who he liked most in the team. 'He makes me look good.'

In recognition of Howe instilling leadership qualities in no single player, it was Dan Burn who later took on the role of changing-room pep-talk giver before the Carabao Cup Final in February 2023, making an impassioned speech and quoting 'Man in the Arena': 'I think I'm a leader, I felt I wanted to say something or I would regret it,' he said before the game. More on that final a bit later.

In an interview to mark the first anniversary of the takeover, Jamie Reuben spoke about what the past 12 months had been like for him and being part of the now awoken Geordie 'sleeping giant', telling NUFC TV:

> It still feels very surreal. Our immediate priority was to restore pride in the club, which I think we have done. I'm predominantly there to support the executive team, I bring ideas and the knowledge of the city. Newcastle is a city I love. The atmosphere five minutes before kick-off at SJP every time still surprises me, it's wonderful to see. Newcastle was a sleeping giant, we're taking a long-term and pragmatic approach, it's exciting. I would like us progressing on every level in the club, performances, style of play – from women's football to the academy, that's the hallmark of success.

Amanda Staveley and Mehrdad Ghodoussi also gave anniversary interviews and equally focused on the positivity of the past 12 months. Amanda said:

> What an incredible year it's been, we're so proud of how far we have come this year. I'm so proud of our women's team, making sure they have the right pathway is critical. Where do we want our women's team to go? To the top! We want them to have the same opportunity as the men. Seeing the excitement of the fans, the community came out to watch them, so excited about Newcastle women. It's been a very humbling experience and the support we had received, from PIF and from the Reuben family and the fans. It's extraordinary, we love what we do.

Mehrad Ghodoussi echoed the importance of the fans in their journey:

> They have been incredible, they are everything as far as we are concerned. They are part of this journey with us, we are family, that's how we look at it. The community is so important to us, it's important to have that connectivity with the city. The success we have had over the past 12 months has been incredible, we have worked as a family and worked as a team and we look forward to the next 12 months, the next five years and the next ten years, and hopefully we will have a lot more success.

The success continued in October with a 0-0 draw against Man Utd, a 1-0 win over Everton and a 2-1 win against Spurs. It was in stark contrast to the tough relegation environment the team were in this time last year, and Wilson was first to admit how the mentality of the team had changed:

> When you're playing you want to be winning games and competing against the best. It's not nice being in a relegation battle and every game is 'must win'. Of course, every game is must win because you want to win, but we're in uncharted territory where the group hasn't been before. So you enjoy the ride rather than feel it's 'must win'. We're putting in solid team performances.

It was time to welcome Villa to St James' Park, right at the end of the month, and also time to welcome more goals for the mighty Toon. Callum Wilson scored a double, with Joelinton and Almirón securing a 4-1 win that saw Newcastle up to fourth place, the hallowed ground of Champions League qualification. If I'm making it seem plain sailing, I apologise. The first half of the game was okay but in the second half they stepped up a gear. Even at 3-0, Howe was urging the team forward for more goals. There was a hunger about the team now and Wilson narrowly missed a hat-trick. It was as if he knew there was an England squad yet to be announced and a national manager looking for impressive strikers to add to his World Cup line-up. Howe acknowledged Wilson's performance:

> I'm really pleased for Callum, the second goal was a typical goalscorer's goal and penalties are never easy. He was at the heart of a lot of our good play today. I'm not too aware what the players know and what they don't know about who comes and who's

> watching them. I almost think it's better that you just play your normal game and you're not overthinking too much. He is, of course, desperate to be involved with England, it's one of his childhood dreams, so he'll be really pleased that he played so well. He scored the two goals and his overall performance was very good.

In the end, Wilson's recent form proved decisive and it was thanks to his three goals in back-to-back matches against Spurs and Villa that he secured his place in the national squad. Or it could have something to do with him visualising and believing in a dream, and never giving up:

> Funnily enough, I was going through my diary the other day, and I'd actually written on today's date (Sunday 13th) – 'Pack for Qatar'. This was probably four months ago I'd written this. I just feel the power of visualisation, that positive affirmation you give with it. That was it. I set my mind to it, to a goal, and I'm so proud of myself. This is just the start, I'm reintegrated back into the squad.

And a few days before the England squad was officially announced, Newcastle consolidated their spot in the top four with another win. Oh, and another four goals. And all on the day before Howe could celebrate his one-year anniversary at the club. Going into the Southampton match so high in the table wasn't a fluke, with only one defeat in the first 13 matches. It was hardly a false position and it was Almirón who started the haul before Chris Wood swivelled sharply and fired into the corner. Willock added a third and Bruno the fourth in a 4-1 victory. Miggy's recent run of goals cemented his improvement under the watchful eye of Howe, who'd instilled confidence in the Paraguay international.

It was a timely show of the positivity that was flowing through the club and the transformation that Howe's leadership had brought to the Tyne – as it stood at this moment in time, he'd won 21 matches from a possible 42 – and his name was being spoken by fans with the same respect they had for the likes of Kevin Keegan and Sir Bobby Robson. The similarities didn't end there either, as in training Howe and his team had created a variety of set-piece routines that would often upset opponents, who thought they'd sussed how the team played, evidenced by the recent 5-1 win over Brentford when Tripps whipped in a corner at pace for Bruno to head home. Or against Villa when Trippier went short again, but found Almirón, who backheeled to find Wilson and a goalscoring header.

There was an excitement to the style of play, usually a 4-3-3 formation, but interchangeable, with the players encouraged to put pressure on defenders while always having an attacking style through a solid midfield and forwards. So no longer was the outlook a stumbling from match to match hoping to stay in the top tier, as now there was a focus and a direction, a purpose and a sense of pride restored. The leaderboards at the training grounds were displayed the week ahead, all mapped out with fixtures and training schedules so every player knew where they stood.

'You won't just see what you're doing, you'll see why you're doing it,' said Ryan Fraser. It was those little things that were making a huge difference. The inside of the training ground, for example, saw a huge change after Howe took over, not just in the structure and look of the place, but the vibe it creates. Motivational signs, such as 'The relentless pursuit of better' and 'Every session, every game, every moment, make it count', created a surge of energy about the place, a far cry from Ashley's décor over a year ago when the crest lay on the floor after falling off the wall.

As starts to the seasons go, there was no doubting the complete reversal this year, and the success continued into November as the team continued their Carabao Cup campaign with a win against Crystal Palace and a 1-0 victory against Chelsea before the World Cup campaign began.

The team got back together just before Christmas for a win against Eddie's former club Bournemouth to take them to the next stage of the Carabao Cup, and whisperings were getting louder that perhaps, just perhaps, there could be some silverware coming our way. To round off the year in the style they'd become accustomed to during this first half of the season, there was a 3-0 victory against Leicester on Boxing Day, with goals from Wood, the ever-reliant Miggy – his ninth goal of the season – and Joelinton. This was a huge match. It had been 45 days since both sides had been in action in the Premier League (and they'd be facing each other in the quarter-finals of the Carabao Cup). It put Newcastle second in the table, a point above Manchester City (who had two games in hand, but who cared?) and seven points off the leaders, Arsenal. The Leicester match was pretty much over in the first half; well, the first 32 minutes to be exact. The King Power Stadium felt the sting of the visitors on form as Chris Wood slotted in a penalty after only three minutes, before Almirón added a second in sublime fashion as he played a lovely one-two with Bruno and then beautifully slotted past Danny Ward on seven minutes. Joelinton headed in the third on 32 minutes from a corner, to allow the Magpies the opportunity to just sit back and enjoy the rest of the Boxing Day game.

Howe was happy with the performance:

> I'd say the performance was up there when you consider the opposition and the game and the break and everything that has gone into to preparing for this game. To start in the manner we did was hugely important. Credit to the players for how they've attacked their game. We scored some very good goals and the general mentality of the group was very, very good after the break. Today was a big test for us and I'm delighted with how the players started.

Second place put Newcastle in a position where they could challenge for the title, but it wasn't something that Howe wanted to get excited about until the time was right:

> I have no problems with the supporters dreaming and talking and speculating about what we can achieve, and no doubt the media will, I can't control that. The only thing we need to be mindful of internally is just focus on what we can control and our own thoughts and actions and how we train and how we prepare. And not look too far ahead and not listen to too much news and media and just focus on our training and make sure we focus on it game by game. This is the toughest league in the world for a reason and our opposition no doubt will be watching us and preparing for us, so we have to be ready.

Finishing the calendar year on 34 points compared to the year before when it was a measly 11 points … Happy New Year to the Toon.

Chapter 10

Gordon, Goals, Going Out

'If he fails, at least he fails while daring greatly, so that his place shall never be with those cold and timid souls who neither know victory nor defeat.'

Roosevelt

'WE HAVE remarkable players, we need a few more remarkable players,' said Amanda Staveley at the beginning of January 2024. It was a bold but true statement. Newcastle had, in the first part of the season, surpassed all expectations. Sitting high in the table, there was a chance to bring in fresh players while the January window was open but, again, because of the FFP restrictions, spending and getting good value for money was proving a problem. As it stood, Newcastle were one of the biggest spenders in the league and, as was known, they couldn't spend more than they earned – the books had to balance. This was tricky as they knew who they wanted to buy, a player they'd had their eye on from last summer, but he was, at the moment, too expensive.

Everton had set a fee of £60m for Anthony Gordon, an amount they'd also asked of Chelsea in the summer.

But the price was too high for Newcastle, so it was a tense first month of the year. Newcastle knew what they wanted but there was a bit of calling of Everton's bluff. They offered £40m plus £5m in add-ons. Everyone held their breath.

'His energy is very high, he's a player I would love to add to the squad,' said Howe, putting more pressure on the club to secure the deal. Happily, as the clock ticked down towards the closing of that 2023 January transfer window, the news broke that 21-year-old Gordon, who'd been with Everton since he was 11 years old, playing at the academy and then at 16 making the first team, was coming to Tyneside. He was very excited, as he confessed:

> It's been a long time coming. I knew the club had been interested in me for a while, I knew in the summer they were interested in me and obviously over the past week it's progressed really quickly. So I'm happy to be here! Since I heard of the interest, I was convinced Newcastle were for me, I think the fanbase and the city suit me as a person, the way the team are playing under the gaffer suits me too. The club just look like they're heading in the right direction and, the way the club's going, I can really excel here.

And the Toon fans were very happy with the signing:

> Rob: I love Anthony Gordon. I was buzzing when we signed him. He's my favourite player. I loved him at Everton, he's a great young player and I always knew he had great potential, and when he was linked with us I was dead happy.

> Alan: I thought Gordon was a good buy. Only recently I think he's come across as a bit lazy at times. He doesn't help out the defence, especially Burn. But he can be very good, he just needs to be more consistent.

Howe was equally excited about his new player:

> I'm delighted to sign Anthony, he's a top, top talent. I'm really excited to work with him, to develop him, and I'm looking forward to seeing what he can do in a Newcastle shirt.

And the manager wasted no time in getting to meet Gordon once he'd been through all the formalities and press calls on his first visit to the club, but, ever the personal manager, football wasn't the subject of conversation, as Gordon revealed:

> We didn't have too much of an in-depth conversation. He was asking about family and how I've been the past few days. Football conversations will come. I'm moving away from my home town, of course, but I'm not nervous about moving to Newcastle. Everyone only has good things to say about Newcastle and the city and I'm getting a bit older and maturing, so it's getting more exciting now and I can't wait to experience the home crowd, I can't wait for the fans to be on my side. It's so hard to come here when you're opposition because St James' Park has the best atmosphere I've ever experienced in England. It's so hard to come here as the away team!

Since he was a child in Everton's academy, Gordon had written down his goals – short-term, medium-term and long-term aims. As a teenager, he spoke in absolutes, with certainty. 'When I play for Real Madrid,' was one example of an initial ambition. Self-belief isn't always easy to come by, indeed perhaps a skill that very few possess and even fewer when you're someone who has to fight for recognition at a young age. At 11, Gordon was rejected by Liverpool and not even quickly snapped up by Everton either, until they reconsidered. Although Everton recognised his attacking talent, there were continuous doubts over his lean physique and his work rate, as David Unsworth, Everton's former academy head and interim manager, explained:

> The biggest problem we had with him was his stamina. So he played a lot of left midfield, on the left of a three, but he would just die on 60 minutes. He would look like he was being lazy and couldn't get back, but it wasn't that, he'd just emptied his tank because he put so much into the first hour.

Clearly a player who was passionate about every game he played in, there was likely to be a little bit of … embarrassment? Is that the right word? Maybe just a bit of 'historical hoo-ha' whenever a player joins a club he has played against previously. Particularly if you're a player who in this case had some heated moments with some of the Magpies in the past:

> It's fine, I've met them all and had a bit of a joke about it. They're fighting for the team, same as me now. I wear my heart on my sleeve and I respect them. I'll always give everything for the badge that

> I'm wearing and I won't apologise for that. I've always said I'll give it my everything.

Meanwhile, my son and others were relieved to hear that Kieran Trippier had signed a new contract in a deal to last until the end of 2023/24 (which was increased in the January transfer window in 2023 until the summer of 2025).

Gordon had a few weeks to get to grips with how things work at the Toon, and was hoping to make his debut against West Ham on 4 February, hinting that he was only just beginning to get going as an international football star:

> I don't think people have seen what I'm capable of yet. My short-term ambitions are to keep winning for the club, keep heading in the right direction. Long term? It has to be trophies.

Talking of trophies, we're going to gloss over the disappointing loss to Sheffield United in the FA Cup and concentrate instead on the Carabao Cup, which saw Newcastle progress to the semi-final stage when they beat Leicester 2-0. Just two days after that other competition loss that we won't mention, St James' Park was now expectant. And they weren't disappointed. It took 60 minutes and several missed chances for the ever-nervous crowd.

> Chris: It felt like we were getting closer and closer and yet we still couldn't score. It was unbelievably nerve-wracking.

But then a goal that, Howe agreed, 'you couldn't script', as local lad Dan Burn got his first for his boyhood club to edge them closer to the semi-final. 'I'm so pleased for him,' said Howe, who cheered alongside the rest of us as the defender ran on to a pass from Joelinton and calmly slotted the ball into the bottom corner. 'This is his club and he has come back here and he's savouring every moment.'

And he did, as Burn explained:

> I used to sit in the East Stand. You always want to score in front of the Gallowgate End. To do that in front of my family was amazing. I like to get forward and it's entertaining watching a guy my size running into the box.

The scoring hadn't finished, however, and to cement the victory came another coolly finished goal, from Joelinton. The St James' Park crowd was delighted. The whisperings of possible silverware were no longer hushed, they roared out of the gates, down the streets, past The Strawberry and infiltrated every part of the city. Newcastle were only one stage away from reaching a final of a cup competition, which they hadn't achieved since 1999. Was it too early to dare to hope?

The small matter of the two-legged semi-final was now the hurdle. Facing Southampton at their home ground on 24 January before welcoming the Saints to St James' Park for the return a week later eked out the excitement, as well as the usual stress, anxiety and tension.

Travelling to St Mary's and backed by 3,200 away fans, Newcastle took to the pitch and within 120 seconds were causing the travelling Toon Army to gasp, cheer and sigh in equal measure when Willock fired over the crossbar and Joelinton had a goal disallowed by the ref, who judged the ball to have hit his arm. Tense wasn't the word. Pope kept out a Southampton chance but it wasn't really too much of a threat to his tenth clean sheet. But if Newcastle were hoping to emulate their 4-1 success against Southampton of the previous year, they weren't quite on track as it was goalless at half-time.

However, the second half finally saw a goal in the 73rd minute, another from Joelinton. Southampton searched for the equaliser and thought they'd succeeded but again the ref saw a hand contact and disallowed the goal. Good decision ref. Then, when Ćaleta-Car took down Saint-Maximin, receiving a second yellow card, any chance of recovery looked pretty bleak for the south coast team with ten men. And it was. Newcastle were one small step closer to the final with this 1-0 victory but now they had to welcome the Saints to St James' Park for the second leg, so it was still all to play for.

You can imagine the media all over the possibility that Newcastle could at last be on track for a trophy, with pundits and commentators all speculating on whether this was the year – as their last major trophy was the Inter Cities Fairs Cup in 1969. Most reckoned it was well overdue.

With a 1-0 advantage from the first leg, Newcastle were aware that Southampton had all the work to do as the whistle blew to start the second leg, but the hosts were buzzing and it was Sean Longstaff who calmed the nerves of the expectant fans with a goal after just four minutes. Yep, the central midfielder took advantage of some impressive work by Tripps, before doing the same again in the 21st minute, putting the Magpies 2-0 up. Although Southampton pulled a goal back, the Longstaff double whammy was the cherry on the cake for the team effort that secured the 3-1 aggregate win, although this was partially tainted by the red card that Bruno received for a challenge on Samuel Edozie. However, getting through to the final of the Carabao Cup was a moment that gave fans hope.

Wearing his black-and-white scarf and waving to fans, newbie Anthony Gordon was watching the game with a smile on his face and soaking up the atmosphere. He looked like he was enjoying every minute of the shouts and cheers from the fans, as if he understood what it meant to every single one of them. Howe, speaking to BBC Radio 5 Live after the game, was ecstatic:

> It feels really good tonight. I'm delighted for everyone connected with the club. It really was a tense night. It was a great atmosphere and brilliant environment for the players to play in.

And what an atmosphere it was. The chants of 'Tell me ma, me ma, we won't be home for tea, we're going to Wembley' rang out around the ground. It rang in the ears of every supporter standing and cheering from their seats, from every hug exchanged and every flag waved. The city was on its feet in celebration and they hadn't even won anything yet. They had, though, in a way, gone one better. The Magpies had ignited the hope and pride back into the city that it could be achieved.

Before the final there were a few league games that the team had to focus on, and first up was a home fixture against West Ham, and Gordon's debut. Coming in midway through the season meant that Howe wanted to ease him in gently, so for 12 appearances he came on as a substitute, his first run-out against the Hammers when he replaced Saint-Maximin. Gordon came out all guns blazing. While he wasn't able to help with the goal haul, Wilson, who hadn't had the best run since coming back from the World Cup, scored Newcastle's only goal. He'd gone 12 games for club and country without a goal so the crowd were up on their feet when it took him just three minutes to find the net.

> Chris: Wilson is a no-frills striker who just gets on with it.

> Henry: I think he's a passionate striker and he rarely misses. You don't always hear much about him when Isak is around.

Although with an early lead things were looking up, West Ham equalised in the first half, so all eyes were on Gordon when he stepped out on the pitch in the 69th minute. The St James' Park faithful made sure they welcomed him in style and there was agreement among the forums that he made a difference in the game by igniting a bit of spirit. Gordon knew he'd be facing competition for a starting spot with Saint-Maximin, Joelinton and, to an extent, Jacob Murphy, but he was keen to prove – as he'd said in his first interview – that people hadn't yet seen what he was capable of.

And he did look capable. He looked bright and showed a spirit and a freshness to get Newcastle on the front foot. He was able to find a rhythm with Wilson and it looked like another goal was on the verge of coming, but it was not to be. The main headline from the game was that Gordon had a lively debut and there was lots of positive passing and movement from a player still so new to the club. Although, in a rather slightly embarrassing moment, fans spotted that he was still wearing his personalised blue-and-white Everton shin pads as he pulled up his socks. He's young. He'll learn.

Shay Given was full of praise for the Gordon cameo and the difference he made towards the end of the game:

> Newcastle – towards the back end, you know the latter part of the game – I think Anthony Gordon made a big difference when he came off the bench, so there's some positives for Eddie Howe not to lose the game. That's important as well, and to keep that unbeaten run going. I suppose such highs in midweek, getting to a Wembley cup final, there's a lot of excitement around the city, but then West Ham, you've got to give them credit as well. A poor start to the game but at the end of the first half and the start of the second half I thought they were the better team. You'd love to have won the game, of course you would, but the lads look a little bit low and a little bit down after the game. But again, it's a point gained on the board.

Fellow Sky Sports pundit Jamie Redknapp was also impressed with Gordon:

> Good debut, really good cameo, he came on and showed what he's about. He's got tremendous pace and he definitely gave them something completely different. They also missed Guimarães in that midfield, he's a really important player in there for them. They miss that quality and they miss that guile when he's not in the team, but it's still an unbeaten run. As disappointing as it'll feel, they're playing so well – it's just the disappointment of not getting the three points that you want.

Redknapp had made the point that others had also noted – the draw was partly down to the absence of Bruno, who played such a crucial part in the team's midfield. Due to his red card against Southampton the closest he got to the action was to watch from the stands, and Howe was equally aware of the Brazilian-sized gap in the team: 'Undoubtedly, he's that difference-maker with an eye for a pass. He has creative flair we possibly missed today.' If you like your stats, this was the fourth Premier League game Bruno had missed this season and Newcastle had failed to win any of them. The fans knew he'd be back for the Carabao Cup Final at the end of the month, but Howe and the team just had to find a way to get some success without him in the matches against Bournemouth and Liverpool before that final.

As it stood, Manchester United had moved into third place in the league table, while Newcastle dropped down to fourth. The worry was that there were so few points between the teams around Newcastle that any poor result could see them fall further away from the top four.

The league games in February weren't anything like those of the first half of the season, with a disappointing 1-1 draw away to Bournemouth and a 2-0 loss at home to Liverpool. The Liverpool game was extra brutal in its scoreline and for the sending off of goalkeeper Nick Pope in the 22nd minute for handling the ball outside the area.

> Chris: What a load of crap that was. There's no way that was a red card, no way; should have been a yellow.

Howe was equally annoyed:

> I think it's harsh, it was a slippery surface and the ball hit the arm; the referee could have given him a yellow card. Nick's very disappointed. He's been magnificent this season and he doesn't deserve to miss next week's game.

Next week's game, of course, being the Carabao Cup Final. Golly gosh, Batman. And it was going to get worse. Martin Dúbravka, Pope's usual deputy, was unable to play, as he was cup-tied after appearing for Man Utd during a loan stint. The previous third choice was Karl Darlow but, having been loaned to Hull in January, he couldn't be recalled. So it was all down to Loris Karius.

Nobody knew how fourth-choice goalie Karius would fare on Sunday, having not played a senior professional game for two years. Nobody was quite sure where his head was at and what battle scars remained after his concussion-induced nightmare in his last appearance for an English club – Liverpool's Champions League Final loss to Real Madrid in 2018. He'd received death threats after that game and he was booed wherever he went.

While Newcastle are quite used to you-couldn't-make-it-up storylines, this redemption arc was a seductive narrative – the potential for one game to change the trajectory of a career forever was something Karius knew only too well. But this is a brutal profession. And the stakes are high and the faith in your own ability and the faith others have in your ability need to be astronomical. And there were many who didn't think this was something he possessed.

'A fourth-choice goalkeeper making his debut in a cup final, when we haven't been to Wembley this century is ridiculous – even by Newcastle's standards!' said fan Walt.

But the ever calm manager, who had no choice with the player he now had in goal, was surely internally – if not outwardly – worried about the lack of recent match action that Karius had to his name. With a week to prepare his team, Howe stressed that they should be looking forward and not back. He didn't want Karius to dwell on his past, but instead to focus on his potential, although you'd probably have to be made of stone to not feel a twinge of panic when he stepped out on the pitch at Wembley. Howe said:

> I've never really discussed it with him at any length. We all have stuff that's happened in our histories, you learn from that, he's no different in that respect. Day one since he's been here, he's been training with our goalkeeper coaches and he's definitely improved, and I think he's in a good place and I think he's ready to play. We have a long build-up to the game, we need to keep our players fresh mentally.
>
> We need to get our preparation right and make sure the players can give their best efforts. You have to look at it as simply another goalkeeper gets an opportunity and we have to be positive. It's exactly why we have a squad of goalkeepers. I have no doubt about his match fitness and I always ask him how he is, and whether we're giving everything he needs to be the best he can be. He's a very likeable laid-back character. I have no doubts of his confidence levels.

Saturday evening on 25 February 2023, and London was awash with black-and-white-adorned fans who braved the trains, the traffic and the London beer prices to get here. Everyone wanted to be here. They'd earned this right, they'd waited for this moment. Newcastle United, without flouting a phrase so flippantly used, were back in the game. There was a host of white smoke guns going up in Trafalgar Square as the good-natured Toon Army, who'd brought with them a whole brigade of fresh recruits that would normally have stayed in their familiar surroundings for the game, were out in force. 'Literally, everywhere I turned there was a black-and-white shirt,' recalled Londoner Nick. 'Every other person that passed me that Sunday lunchtime was in a Newcastle shirt. I do travel a lot and at one point I genuinely wondered if I'd woken up in the wrong city.'

A dream had partly come true and that dream was on the brink of becoming a heavenly reality for those that had travelled south to witness their team take part in their first final since 1999 and, at that point, there was an air of peace over the crowds. 'At that point, I remember getting off the tube on the walk up to Wembley and thinking it didn't matter if we won or we lost, we'd been noticed again,' recalled supporter Shaz. 'I know it sounds weird to say and of course I wanted to win, but I was going to Wembley for heaven's sake, to watch Newcastle play in a final. I felt in a way I'd already won!'

I didn't ask her if that sentiment still held true 90 minutes later when the game was all over. But I understood. The team and the fans felt like they were on the brink of lots of these finals to come. So, whatever happened, this wasn't a fluke, this wasn't a 'we won't get this chance again for a while' occasion, and therefore there was a lack of pressure from the fans. But on the flip side of that, of course, was that there was a 68-year domestic trophy itch they were desperate to scratch. The trophy drought had long become hard to bear. 'I don't know what I'd do if we won and we finally had a trophy …' said Olly. 'I think I'd have to get me ma to slap us or something to check it worn't a dream.'

Pre-kick-off there was no doubting the Geordie presence. The Newcastle end was packed in a well-orchestrated display, and black-and-white flags were waving frantically, manically, expectantly. The other half of the stadium didn't seem half as fussed, the red shirts slowly ambling in without voice or coordinated displays of fanfare.

> Steve (who'd travelled down to Wembley in a ten-hour car journey two days before): We made sure we weren't going to let the team down when they'd done so much for us; we were ready. I don't care how long you've not been to a final, you give it your all as a supporter every time. It just seemed to me that Man U fans had been to finals a lot more than us. Me, I was dead happy to be here; some of them didn't look to be bothered!

The ones that didn't look that bothered could well have been Trippier's family, the England player admitting that all his family are Red Devils fans!:

> Me dad, me brothers, they're all Reds. I hope they support me. I tried to get them tickets, I hope I've got enough. And, yes, I've got them tickets for the Newcastle end. My brothers and my mates, we've had a bit of banter but of course they're fully behind me.

In a way, whatever happened on the pitch, the mood didn't change for the crowd. Allan Saint-Maximin gave them the biggest cause for hope when, 32 minutes into the game, his strike was saved by David de Gea. And then it was Manchester United's Casemiro who achieved the not insignificant feat of getting between Schär and Botman to power home the Red Devils' first goal. Six minutes later Rashford looped a shot over Karius's outstretched hands. He couldn't react in time, and it was 2-0 to the Reds.

Howe went for broke at the start of the second half, introducing Alexander Isak up front alongside Callum Wilson. Newcastle needed something. There was little to fault in Newcastle's effort or strategy here. But Manchester United had seized control towards the end of the first half, and the gulf in big-match expertise was soon apparent. Of the Newcastle starting XI only Bruno had won a final of consequence – although Trippier and Botman had won league titles, with Atlético Madrid and Lille respectively. For everyone else, this was new territory. Even Blyth-born Burn, in the week before the game, admitted how relaxed he felt about the situation – and he should be the one to feel the weight of expectation the most. He'd given a rousing speech before the match in the dressing room and read aloud 'The Man in the Arena', which was written by Theodore Roosevelt in April 1910. It was an emotional reading, and watching it back on the Amazon Prime documentary in which it featured brought a tear to my eye:

> It is not the critic who counts; not the man who points out how the strong man stumbles, or where the doer of deeds could have done better. The credit belongs to the man who is actually in the arena, whose face is marred by dust and sweat and blood; who strives valiantly; who errs, who comes short again and again, because there is no effort without error and shortcoming; but who does actually strive to do the deeds; who knows great enthusiasm, the great devotions; who spends himself in a worthy cause; who at the best knows in the end the triumph

> of high achievement, and who at the worst, if he fails, at least fails while daring greatly, so that his place shall never be with those cold and timid souls who neither know victory nor defeat.

At half-time, even 2-0 down, there was still plenty of hope – even trying to defend against a team with half a billion pounds worth of attacking talent. Newcastle had seen plenty of the ball, won plenty of duels, created plenty of little half-openings. It was enough to keep the game alive for those watching.

> Chris: We're going to win this, that's all I kept thinking. We'd been playing so well before all this, we'd only lost once in something like 20 games and even that was from a lousy eighth-minute extra-time goal.

> Henry: When we went 1-0 I was heartbroken. With no Nick Pope, I wasn't confident in Karius. But then, saying that, his second goal was very unlucky and he made lots of good saves; you can't blame him for it.

Even though Newcastle continued to fight, attack after attack was broken down and, in the end, when the final whistle blew, their wait for silverware continued.

Chairman Yasir Al-Rumayyan and Amanda Staveley applauded politely from the royal box but they could see the potential – the team they'd taken on over a year ago that were destined for relegation that season were now at Wembley and had lost in a cup final. That's a considerable achievement, whichever way you look at it.

Chapter 11

Champions *Whisper* League

'I'm not focusing on the league table but I do know we won again and that's the main thing.'

Eddie Howe

MARCH CAME with a spring in its step and the Carabao Cup a distant memory. Well, not quite, it was still early days and the defeat still felt raw. But it doesn't do to dwell on things and, in the words of Eddie Howe, you pick yourself up and you carry on. It felt a little harsh that the first match after their cup final defeat was an away game at Manchester City, the team who were fighting for top spot and the league title race entering its defining phase.

Eddie Howe had stated that he wanted Newcastle to show early intent and they'd listened to the gaffer. There was no woeful or lacklustre display – quite the opposite, in fact. Bruno lifted Toon Army spirits early on by spinning the ball in behind Kyle Walker to Anthony Gordon, who was making his full debut. It didn't go quite to plan, though, and Gordon, to the home crowd's glee, kicked his own foot instead. It was another opportunity for dusting down and cracking on mentally but, while that was happening, Foden was putting one past Nick Pope for the opening goal.

But there were still plenty of signs of life in the Geordie attack – Callum Wilson and Sean Longstaff both had good chances in the first half but neither could quite cross the line. It's fair to say Newcastle were causing plenty of problems for City and causing quite a threat when Allan Saint-Maximin, Joe Willock and Isak were all introduced at the same time, just after the hour mark. City looked under threat at times, and even scrappy, but then substitute Bernardo Silva slotted home to put the game out of the Magpies' reach midway through the second half.

'It felt like we were playing chase ball,' said fan George. 'We're making plenty of chances but not quite getting the goals. We don't want to start forgetting how to score this stage in the league.'

The win meant that City moved to within five points of Arsenal, while Newcastle remained in fifth place, four points behind Tottenham.

Although the result was disappointing, there were positives to take from the loss. Isak was back to full fitness and looked ready to do some damage whenever he got the ball, and the team's spirit never seemed to dwindle. They simply acknowledged that they were playing with the big boys now and were just about holding their own. For Howe, there were plenty of positives, even though they'd only (whisper it) won one of their past eight league games:

> I thought they played really well, it was very good performance from us. We were brave and we unsettled them, we had our moments but we weren't as clinical as them. Our general performance we have to be positive about. We're trying to be the team we

> want to be in every game. We hurt them at times but couldn't put that final piece together; Joelinton's chance at 1-0 sticks in my head. You need to be clinical with your chances because you're not going to get many, and unfortunately that didn't happen. We want to be aggressive and progressive, and there are still areas to get better in, but the overall feeling leaving here is very positive.

If you need a bit of positivity in your life, then chances are a home game will lift your spirits. And it certainly did on 12 March when Newcastle welcomed Wolves to St James' Park. The home crowd were roaring and clapping in excitement from the moment the whistle blew and there were plenty of oohs and aahs all round the stadium, as the Magpies looked like the dominant team they should be. Isak didn't disappoint them. There's no secret that the fans love an attacking style of play, one that's strong, brave and direct, and Isak gave it to them in abundance. After his goal put Newcastle ahead, the crowd seemed mesmerised by his every touch. It was a proper, old-fashioned centre-forward's goal – space, timing and athleticism to make the perfect connection – and it was also the team's first goal since the beginning of February.

Howe said of Isak:

> Hopefully this is the start of a really good spell for him. He's capable of everything a centre-forward needs. He has pace, technique and strength and that's why the goal pleased me. I think he's capable of great things and it's up to us to keep him in a good place and feed him in the right areas.

Speaking before the game, Howe said he hoped for a 'spark or individual moment' to get the team's flagging season back on track, and Isak heard the call and answered tenfold. When he came off midway through the second half after signalling that he was exhausted, the whole crowd were on their feet cheering the player who'd run, run and run some more. I mentioned to my husband that he seems like a player who's a lot stronger than he looks, not to mention one helluva quick runner.

And talking of speed, after Wolves had equalised there was a need for a new hero to come to the forefront to make sure that Newcastle didn't come away with just another draw. And that new hero came in the shape of – who else? – Almirón. Celebrating his 11th goal of the season, Almirón, who'd come on with just 20 minutes left, gave the crowd a reason to lift the roof off St James'. The poor run would have stretched to one win in seven if Wolves had secured a draw, but it didn't, and the Magpies got their deserved three points. It underlined their European credentials, lifting them back above Liverpool into fifth and just four points below Tottenham with two games in hand. A 2-1 victory was theirs, the points were theirs, the Champions League spot could still be theirs.

Howe told Sky Sports after the game:

> The first-half performance in general was very good. Alexander Isak scored a massive goal for us. When it's a one-goal lead, it's very delicate. It should have been more at half-time. Wolves came back into the game, but the character shown by the group to go again and get the winning goal is a great feeling for us.

My husband was full of praise for Miggy.

> Chris: Almirón, he's grown into such a good player, he's naturally very quick but couldn't finish to begin with. And then all of a sudden he'd find a way to get in behind the defence and score. And he'd do this all the time, it was absolutely brilliant.

It felt like a lot more than a 2-1 victory – it was a victory for Newcastle's spirit and, above all, testament to their strength of character. Talking of which, the Magpies were tested when they travelled to Nottingham Forest just five days later and managed to come from behind to secure another 2-1 win. It was the first time this season they'd won from being behind but not the first time that the goalscoring hero was Isak. The Swedish striker cancelled out Emmanuel Dennis's opener in the first half to bring the Magpies level. And while there were plenty of chances for Newcastle to take the lead, including Elliot Anderson thinking he'd made it 2-1 when he thumped in a header at the back post, only for it to be ruled out by VAR for offside in the build-up, it wasn't until stoppage time, when a handball by Niakhaté was penalised, that Isak stepped forward to take and score the winning penalty.

Howe said afterwards:

> There was a lot in that game, it was action-packed. I think we were the dominant team, we didn't deserve to go behind, and I'm delighted to win, it's a massive three points. Whenever you come back is hugely satisfying. Our general play is very good. There was a spell in the first half, for about 15 minutes, where

> we lost our focus, we became a bit emotional, we let the crowd get into the game. The goal rocked us but apart from that we created chances. There was a lot of character shown in the group. Alex is our designated penalty taker and he did what he had to do. Two wins back to back, we needed it. It was a difficult experience, the cup final, because we were desperate to win.

Travelling supporters remained packed in the stands long after the final whistle, celebrating with the players on the pitch and chanting for their success in what could prove to be a significant result. Howe was keen to acknowledge that, yet again, the travelling fanbase played a huge part in securing their win:

> The fans never disappoint, they were a feature in the game, which is unusual for the away crowd. They kept with us, they kept going and in the end they made the difference.

These three points meant that Newcastle were just a point behind Tottenham with a game in hand. It also meant that, despite the prediction at the start of the season for Newcastle to hit the heady heights of eighth or even seventh place, the Magpies were flying higher.

Shakespeare once wrote that 'April hath put a spirit of youth in everything', and that was certainly true for Newcastle, who managed a phenomenal sprightly haul of 22 goals in the month. Despite April being the penultimate month of the season, because of the World Cup break in December, and an international break at the end of March, Newcastle still had 31 per cent of their league campaign to play. Which meant they had seven games in April and another five in May.

It was the time that all could have been lost in the final stages of the race for the top four, yet the Magpies stepped up a gear and showed they were very much, in the words of Elton, 'still standing' when their first game came, against their Carabao Cup Final victors Man Utd. If there was a doubt that the loss lingered in the St James' Park changing rooms, it was quickly extinguished when the hosts battered the Red Devils 2-0 on 2 April, a win that seemed to set the standard for the rest of the month.

In front of a buoyant St James' Park, the Magpies not only beat Man Utd but went above them into third place, a position that they maintained for the next 30 days. And they could have recorded even more goals thanks to the persistence and hunger of the players out on the pitch. Willock and Isak both went on the attack but were denied, the former trying again before it was third time lucky when he cemented the first goal in front of a jubilant home crowd that had been on and off their feet in excitement. Callum Wilson, who came on as a sub, doubled the team's haul in the 88th minute, possibly fuelled by the cup final defeat, which had 'left a sour taste', as he said after the victory:

> We had to put it right in front of our fans. Now we're starting to find a bit of momentum. There are some big games coming up. It's about being consistent. There's still a very long way to go. There will be a lot of twists and turns until the end of the season. Today we gave ourselves the best opportunity to get third and progress up the table.

Dan Burn was in agreement, telling Sky Sports:

> Over the seasons we've always wanted to beat Man Utd. It's really special. For a long time we've always disliked Man Utd as Newcastle fans. We owed them one this season. It was good to get a win.

Howe was also keen to impress the idea that the energy and the fitness the team displayed should hopefully keep them in good stead for the rest of the busy month:

> It was an important win. We had high energy and there were lots of chances created. We kept knocking on the door, and that's a tribute to our fitness levels today; in my opinion we got stronger. We're a team full of really good athletes, we play a high-energy, high-pressing style, something that we consistently work on in training and it paid dividends today.

Former Newcastle winger Chris Waddle was especially impressed by his old club:

> Newcastle have been cheered on by a very passionate crowd and they deserved to win. Losing a cup final hurts but they've turned up, worked their socks off and said, 'We're not being beaten.' We've seen a glimpse this season of what it would be like, should Champions League football return here. They've got the momentum and the fans, so they have it all going on. The attitude in this Newcastle squad shows they're on a mission.

It was a sentiment shared by Shay Given:

> It's a massive result. It's a special day for these fans – hopefully they can get the job done. I'm sure revenge was part of the team talk. These are special times for them. Eddie Howe deserves such credit.

Talking of revenge, Henry went to school the following day itching to see his best friend Rory, the Manchester United fan who'd watched the Carabao Cup Final with him only a few weeks before.

Three days later the Toon were back in action again, travelling to the Hammers for an evening kick-off and hopes of another win – they had ten away Premier League wins over the London side already – and win they did, in style. Harping back to the first half of the season when they were winning by a handful of goals, the Magpies beat West Ham 5-1, with two goals from Wilson, two from Joelinton and one from Isak.

Wilson, it has to be said, must love coming up against West Ham. He'd scored 12 times in his previous 13 appearances against them and, due to his previous success, he told *Footballers' Football* podcast that he'd do the Macarena in celebration if he scored again. And, of course, when he found himself unmarked 12 yards out to head in the first goal of the game, he did indeed show the stadium his moves.

Newcastle's second goal saw Fabian Schär beat the whole back line with a long ball that reached Joelinton, and while his goal was initially flagged offside, a VAR check confirmed that the Magpies were 2-0 up. The Hammers roused a little at that point, frustratingly for Pope, and they scored from a corner just before half-time. But that slight glimmer wasn't enough to slow down the Magpie machine, and, just seconds into the second half, Murphy stole the ball from Fabianski and passed to Wilson to tap in. No Macarena at that point, but the huge smile said it all. There were no such smiles from the Hammers' defence when the fourth goal from Newcastle saw the keeper miscontrol a long ball after running out of goal, leaving Isak aiming for an empty net to make it five. Thank you and goodnight.

As usual, Howe was calm and controlled:

> It was a strange scoreline but we scored some great goals, and when we clicked into gear we were very good. Really good performance from Callum, I was really pleased with his first goal. He was where he needed to be in the first goal, and the second goal I didn't think he could miss, and very unselfish from Jacob. He's a real outstanding goalscorer and a huge player for us. I was pleased with the second half. I think we played with more control. I think from the high on Sunday and the quick turnaround in games, it was always going to be a challenge but I felt we dealt really well with that.

The quick turnaround in games continued, as three days later Newcastle were away at Brentford, and faced a tough game against the Bees. The hosts wasted no time in exerting a slice of dominance over Newcastle, who failed to muster a single shot on target in a lacklustre first-half display. Newcastle played in the customary 4-3-3 but they were struggling to get into the game, with Brentford successful in their numerous set pieces and corners. Newcastle were eventually punished when they gave away two penalties. The first came after Botman barrelled into Kevin Schade in the 29th minute, but Pope produced a wonderful dive to save the penalty. However, Brentford's second was successful, Toney converting to make it 1-0 in added time of the first half. There was a lot of speculation at half-time that the Magpies' winning streak might be coming to an end. But these people underestimated the half-time team talk, and whatever Howe said clearly worked.

Newcastle came out with an energy and intensity that had been lacking, as well as a change of formation, as Howe deployed a two-striker system, bringing on Anthony Gordon and Callum Wilson. The Magpies levelled the score after 54 minutes thanks to the Brentford goalkeeper, who diverted the ball into his own net from Joelinton's across-the-goal strike. Then it was Isak who put the Toon ahead seven minutes later when he curled his shot into the top corner from the edge of the box after Wilson had rolled the ball to him on the edge of the area. Wilson coming on seemed to ignite Isak, who looked the quality signing the travelling Toon fanbase had come to appreciate more and more. But they also saw a team come back from falling behind, a team with a strength and mentality to fight back and a team that, again, had kept their winning momentum going strong.

'That was a really tough game, the players looked totally exhausted,' said Wills. 'Eddie must be a miracle worker. I don't know how exactly he got us out of that trap, but in terms of coaching was a masterpiece.'

> Grampy: Three games in six days and three wins … I don't think the fans could believe it.

There was a slight bit of drama on the touchline, however, when Howe, who brought on Gordon in the second half, subbed him off again for Matt Targett with seconds to go. Gordon wasn't impressed and shoved Howe's hand away when he trudged off the pitch, seemingly frustrated at the gaffer's decision to bring him off. Howe was keen to play down the event; he didn't want to create a drama that the press were seemingly eager for, especially as his new player had been, in the past, known to be reactive. 'He's obsessed with being the best; it physically hurts him if he hasn't been the best in training,' said a member of Gordon's tight-knit inner circle, speaking anonymously to protect their relationship. 'He has that personality. Everything's a game. Everything he has to win.'

It was a sentiment shared by David Unsworth, talking of his experience with Gordon at Everton:

> The biggest thing for me was that he was always searching to go to the next level early. At under-16s, he was desperate to get into the under-18s. As soon as he was in the under-18s, he was trying desperately to come with me [in the under-23s]. As soon as he came with me, he was desperate to get into first-team training. That desire to get to the next level is something you can't really instil in people.

Howe knew that this strong personality trait might need harnessing but he accepted that Gordon was overly emotional:

> Part of me understood why he acted like he did. I didn't condone it. You don't want to see any player react like that because, suddenly, you'll have a team that looks like it doesn't have the discipline that it needs.
>
> I made a decision based on Anthony going down holding his ankle, based on the fact there were

> seconds left on the clock, to try and do what I felt I needed to do to win the game. He needed to accept that and, if he had an issue, come and see me in private. That's how I felt he should have reacted in that situation, but it's a young player learning about the game and learning about us at the same time. I've got no issue with him.

One of Howe's 'non-negotiables', of course, is that his players put the interests of the team first and that this solidarity had been a key part of the team's rise to third place. And just like Gordon, when he arrived in January, any new arrivals the club might acquire in the summer would be immersed in that mentality:

> We've had success this year based on that one principle: the team is the most important thing. Of course, we want individuals within the team to excel and have great seasons, and a number of players have, but never at the expense of the team. That has to be at the forefront of the players' minds.

Howe was eager to add that Gordon's passion was something that should be harnessed, but used when playing football rather than off the pitch:

> His enthusiasm, aggression and motivation are high. He's determined to do well and achieve. It's a hallmark of his, and we love that. In certain moments he needs a cool head. You want good people off the pitch, good pros living their life right, and on the pitch lads who want to win, passionate about what they're doing. Take that away and he's not the same

> player. Just needs a bit of refining around the edges. When he came on he changed the game for us. He accepted he was overly emotional, we moved on very quickly and had a 10 to 15 minute conversation, where it's really important that I help him. He's a young player. He has so much talent and ability but he needs help to get to where his career should go. Fingers crossed we can work on that together.

Interestingly, in an interview with the *Daily Mail* in March 2024, a year after the event, Gordon recalled the impact of having a calming and undramatic manager in charge, one who leads by example with his behaviour. If Howe was throwing boots and shouting and yelling unapologetically, it would lead to similar disruptive behaviour among the team. This was not the Newcastle way. Gordon said of the incident, having apologised that April afternoon but then having had a couple of days before he saw the gaffer again:

> The way the manager handled it, that helped me so much. We had two days off after and I just remember the anxiety. Nothing could get rid of it. I couldn't really go about my day. I was horrendous company for my family. It was that sick feeling in my stomach. I'm passionate, but that was way overstepping the mark. Honestly, the days off killed me! Someone texted saying: 'Are you training with the under-23s?' I'm thinking, *What? No one has told me so, but am I?* I spoke to the gaffer as soon as I came back in. I was so surprised at how he handled me. He basically said, 'Whether you like it or not, you're going to be a success here.' I did not expect that conversation. He understood where I was coming

> from. It was the insecurity of not doing what I thought I would. I regret it, of course.

That moment of regret, however, would find itself turning into an advantage – perhaps lessons learned about conduct are best learned the hard way. A few weeks later, when the team played against Brighton, Gordon rushed over to celebrate the opening goal with his team-mates even though he wasn't playing at the time. It was testament to everything Howe and the management team lived by. 'I want us to be relentless in the pursuit of winning. A team determined to win and do everything they can.' Howe's words, spoken only seven days previously, now seemed a little hollow as the team came off the pitch at Villa Park, utterly defeated – mentally and literally – having lost 3-0. It was their fourth match of the month and they had three more to play in April, which meant that they had to very quickly and successfully shake off this defeat. But easier said than done, right? Especially when Aston Villa moved to within six points of the Magpies after their victory. It was a sobering defeat for Newcastle and, as Howe later revealed, it was their worst performance of the season:

> Sometimes these things, when they happen, it can be a good thing because it just reminds everyone of the fragility of performance. The main focus is on what our response will be. We need to make sure we're not that team again. It's just a disappointing day, one we have to analyse, but put to bed quickly. At this stage of the season with so few games to go you have to focus on what's ahead rather than what's gone. It was a tough afternoon. But the lads

> have been so consistent through the season. These things can happen. We just now need to focus on the response.
>
> In all disciplines we were slightly off our best and we were punished by a very good team. In every aspect it was unlike us, we were wasteful with the ball, and out of possession we weren't as solid and tight as we have been. I've spoken with the players and given my feelings. We weren't ourselves, we didn't represent ourselves in the way we can. That is the first time it's happened in a long time. Today we were just a level off.

Howe's frustration was probably slightly elevated due to the manager he lost to – Unai Emery:

> Without a doubt it was [a life-changing moment]. I'm here because Unai turned the job down, so I'm delighted that he did! Fate has a strange way of working and now we come together.

And speaking of together, the team mentality mirrored Howe's, with Trippier also keen to forget this lunchtime loss, speaking to BT Sport:

> From minute one we knew we weren't right. Aston Villa came out of the traps quickly. The way we played wasn't ourselves. We've got to forget about this result as we have big games coming up. Like I said before, out of possession we're normally aggressive and press. Today in possession we were long ball and that's unlike us. We will focus on the game against Spurs.

With seven days to come together and regroup, the focus in training for the upcoming Tottenham game was simple: to win. The home fans heard the call and were ready to help them on their way to victory, although I doubt even a betting man would have taken on the odds of the Toon winning 6-1. Or that they'd score five of those goals in the first 21 minutes of the game!

The sense of expectation in the air was heavier than usual because of the loss the week before and the teetering of the team in the Champions League qualifying positions. The Magpies, inspired by an electric atmosphere, started hard and fast, taking just 62 seconds to open the scoring. And from that point onwards, they didn't give Spurs a minute's peace.

The first goal came from a player previously described as being on the 'periphery' of the team but who Howe now credits with being 'a key member of his side'. Joelinton drove inside from the edge of the box and his low ball fell into the path of Murphy, who was there to smash it in. The latecomers to the game had barely a chance to sit down before they were up again cheering. 'It's not often you have a start like that in a game,' said Howe. 'Especially one of such importance. Jacob has grown into the team, he's got a lot of qualities, he can play various positions and he took his goals very well today.'

Note that all-important plural when talking about Murphy's goals. But we'll come to that. Hold on to your hats, as five minutes later it was Joelinton who rounded Lloris to double the lead. It was while the home fans were celebrating goal number two that Murphy decided it was time for another and rattled in a third with a curling shot that Lloris didn't even bother to try to reach. Perhaps he couldn't quite keep up with what was going on, as there was definitely an air of 'we can't catch our breath, are we actually 3-0 up with only nine minutes played?!'

> Chris: Murphy is incredibly quick. He injects a different energy, a different pace when he's playing. He's a fantastic utility player who has the capability of playing different positions but brings fantastic attributes from the bench.

> Henry: He's very funny too, Dad, he's cheeky. He's got a lot of skills and he knows when to pass the ball. Some players don't always know when to pass.

Not wanting to miss out on any of the scoring action, Isak decided the time was right to start his goal haul. After Willock delivered a sumptuous ball in, Isak looked like he was playing in a leisurely Sunday league match as he calmly slotted the ball home. And if Spurs fans were already sinking low in their seats, they sank even lower (let's face it, some were even heading back to the Metro station for the train home) when Isak pummelled another goal from a tight angle and Lloris did actually try to save it this time.

When the half-time whistle blew there was almost an audible sigh of relief from the Spurs players, who looked as shell-shocked as the Toon Army were delirious. Harry Kane did prevent it being a complete whitewash when a few minutes into the second half he pulled one back. But Wilson, who'd replaced Isak and also wanted a bit of action, took a pass from fellow sub Almirón to take the scoreline to 6-1.

> Henry (who could recall exactly where he was as the match played out): I couldn't believe it. I was out

> in the woods with Uncle Matt and his phone kept tinging. He kept saying to me, 'First goal, Henners.' Then a few minutes later, 'Another goal,' and then literally a few minutes later, 'Another one, Henry!' I thought he was winding me up till I got home and saw you, Mum.

'That's the reaction we wanted,' said Howe, albeit his comment not about Henry, more on the team:

> It was an incredible start to the match from us. I thought we were very good. The crowd were incredible for us and we elevated our performance during that opening half an hour. You're planning during the week on how you're going to impose yourselves on your opponents. I think the big message was for us to play our game as we don't think we did against Aston Villa. I said before the game that it was about realigning our principles of play. We planned as if they might change [to a back four]. We thought it was a realistic possibility so we worked on that in the week, and it's all about being adaptable in the Premier League. We want the high energy and intensity off the ball and then we want the calmness on it. We want progressive football so the lads have had to take on a lot of information but they're doing incredibly well. Since I walked through the door here, the players have responded so well to us and I can't thank them enough really.

Howe still wouldn't be drawn on whether his team would be in the top four by the end of May:

> It's not for me to say. I saw a very good team playing today, but there's a lot of games to go and a lot of points to play for.

Whereas Tripps, speaking to Sky Sports, was ready to make that prediction and wanted to say the words Champions League and Newcastle in the same sentence:

> We shouldn't be scared to say we want to play Champions League football. We knew how big it was against Tottenham. Thc games are now running out but we've got another one around the corner so we need to be ready for that.
>
> This club and this stadium would be bouncing if we could bring Champions League football back here. The gaffer has put faith in the players here. They've shown how good they are. The fans have been unbelievable all season. Since I've arrived, they've been incredible, home and away. The results have obviously helped, but hopefully that can continue. Newcastle and Atlético have the best supporters I've ever played for, but Newcastle take it up to another level.

With two more games to play in seven days – away to Everton and then home to Southampton on the last day of the month – you'd be forgiven for thinking that any lesser team would be on their knees. But there was no let-up for their opponents, who were about to face a fired-up Magpies who were following a dream.

Chapter 12

Bad Times Don't Last but Legends Do

'I told me wife I'd be at the departures lounge if she needed me.'

Jeff

WHILE EDDIE Howe wanted to keep focused on each game and not think about the 'what if' situation, it seemed every other Geordie fan in the entire country was doing the overthinking for him.

'We know why Eddie didn't want to count his chickens but we were so close … it was probably reassuring not to have a manager who was thinking it was "a given" that we'd finish in the top four. We had a calming captain at the helm, he'd tell us when it was time,' said Kev.

'Nope, we were in the Champions League, no doubt about it mate, we were there,' Tim argued. 'Barring a colossal late-season collapse, we'll be back to the Champions after 20 years!'

'I had me passport updated and at the ready,' remembers fan Jeff. 'I said to me wife I'd be at the departures lounge if I could right now!'

If you were a Newcastle fan that needed more of a hint that their team would be enjoying Champions League football next season, it came in their last two games of April. An away match at Goodison Park not only saw the mighty Toon win 4-1 but Wilson continue to add to his record goalscoring haul. If they were on a high with another prolific win, you should spare a thought for Everton, who faced their 17th demoralising defeat of the season.

Wilson opened the scoring for the visitors in the 28th minute with an instinctive finish. The in-form Joelinton added to the tally and Newcastle showed their strength in depth as Isak eluded several challenges with some sensational dribbling – it's worth watching this on YouTube as the way he moves with a ball is just mind-blowing – to set up an easy finish for fellow sub Murphy at the far post. Wilson's second goal, in the 75th minute, was a tremendous strike, curling a finish past the reach of England goalkeeper Jordan Pickford. This was his eighth goal in the last six games against the Toffees.

It could have been worse for Everton but Pickford managed to brilliantly tip away a Willock volley, and defender Fabian Schär was denied a late goal when it was ruled offside. Much earlier, Dominic Calvert-Lewin thought he'd made it 1-1 on the stroke of half-time, but it was ruled offside. Everton did manage to claw one goal back, which went in directly from a corner kick, but it made no difference, especially against a Magpies team that had been prolific in front of goal and were a well-drilled, well-organised outfit. It was another emphatic victory, their seventh in eight games but, for Everton, the danger of it being something of a last hurrah in the Premier League. Howe was very pleased:

> It's a return to goalscoring ways in the last few games, which is great to see. We scored some great goals. I think we were solid defensively, we knew there would be an aerial challenge. We were a bit bitty with the ball in the first half but second half we put our foot to the floor. Callum's goals were great to see. First goal, typical goal from him, second one spectacular, great to see at such a crucial moment. The build-up, Isak created a piece of skill. He's got incredible ball manipulation.

When asked about the third position that Newcastle had been sitting in for the last month and looked set to remain in, it was no surprise that Howe wouldn't be drawn into a definitive answer:

> I have not commented on the top four, I'm just focusing on the next game in the league. We've got a quick turnaround with Southampton. We have two days to prepare, which will be a difficult game, so the end table will tell us where we are, but at the moment I'm just concentrating on the next game. We know nothing is taken for granted from our perspective. It puts us in a lot stronger position. To get six points from Tottenham and Everton is a great return.

Everton manager Sean Dyche summed it up perfectly afterwards: 'Newcastle are free-rolling. They're flying.'

So the Magpies flew on to their last game of April, a home fixture against Southampton, and one that this author and her family travelled up to see. Henry and Chris got the honours of watching the game and reporting back to me while I spent the next 90 minutes soaking up the atmosphere with my other two children and doing a bit of shopping. Trying to explain to the train conductor that we were coming up from the south but didn't support Southampton, we were going to watch Newcastle, who we did support, provided at least half an hour of entertaining conversation. And the moment we arrived at the train station in Newcastle, it felt like we'd come home. There was an air of excitement as we made our way along the River Tyne and up the hill towards our hotel, the excitement increasing as we headed to The Strawberry, where we enjoyed a game of pool. The number of games increased when we started chatting to the locals, who kept paying for us to play because 'you're here to enjoy yourselves, we want ya to have a fun time!'

There was such a collective feeling of camaraderie, and Henry soaked up all the photos, the posters, the memorabilia that was on display. We wandered slowly around the perimeter of the stadium, posing by Shearer's statue and reading Robson's epitaph. We imagined that we were players coming in and up the steps for the first time and we glimpsed the green pitch through the steel gates. It was heaven drenched in black and white and we hadn't even watched the game yet.

> Henry: When we were walking up to the game, there was a drummer playing. Dad and I could hear him and there was just like a general noise of people all excited. We saw someone selling hats, and Dad bought me one. The atmosphere, even walking up the road by the Gallowgate End, it was like a tunnel and it was so noisy but in a good way. It was so loud, even hours before the game, there was lots of singing. No one was in a bad mood even when we went 1-0

> down. Everyone was shouting and standing up and everyone was singing, and so even though we were behind, it was still positive.
>
> There was a man behind me who said to me, 'Don't worry, we're going to win this game, we're going to win big.' I think he thought Dad and I were worried. I was worried. I might have been bad luck as they'd been winning every game and now we were losing. But when Wilson scored we were up jumping and laughing, and when we scored the second and the third, we did the same. We had another chance right before the end, it was such a good game.
>
> Everybody said hi to you as you walked past, everyone in the stadium or walking back from the game. There was a guy sitting next to me and we were chatting, and I didn't know him and we shook hands. I found a flag too. They were laid down on the concrete slabs before us. There was a couple who had one in front of them and I asked them if I could have it, and they said, 'Yeah sure, enjoy the game!' I swear I nearly hit Dad about five times with the corner bit of the flag.

Memories like this will stay with my son forever, something I'm very grateful to everyone at St James' Park for.

But back to football. There was a surprising start to the match in that Saints opened the scoring, with Armstrong giving the away fans something to cheer about. And let's face it, they hadn't had much of that recently as they were currently sitting six points adrift at the bottom of the table. But they only had about 13 minutes (plus half-time) to celebrate before Wilson, coming on as a sub for the second half, decided that he hadn't finished adding to his impressive goal tally. He scored from a free kick nine minutes into the second half. Howe had decided to keep him on the bench initially, but after a disappointing first half he brought on his main goalscorer and the game changed pretty quickly.

Seeing Wilson run on was probably the point that it all started to look ominous for the Saints fans, who'd have been well aware that once Wilson had a taste for a goal, he'd be hungry for more. And he was, rounding the goalkeeper in a display of great composure to slot in his second. But before that – and we're sorry to bring it up, Saints – an own goal by Theo Walcott had already cemented their misery. Wilson nearly had a third in the dying seconds of the game but he hit the bar. However, none of the Newcastle faithful were complaining. We could hear the cheers as we came out of the Metrocentre, a brief respite from shopping and chance to get some fresh air, the sound of celebrations filling the air.

Eddie Howe said after the match:

> [It was a] much better display in the second half, we knew it was going to be a tough game, we knew Southampton's qualities. Callum was outstanding, he's a brilliant player to have in our squad. He's always had the desire to score, every game, every training session, it's great to see him getting the rewards that his performances deserve. It's a tough league and we will have tough games to come. We'll enjoy the momentum; I can't thank the supporters enough.

There was just a week to prepare before the Arsenal game, which kicked off the final month of the season, in which Newcastle had five matches to play. The Gunners' boss, Mikel Arteta, admitted that his team were full of motivation after suffering defeat last time they played the Magpies at the end of the previous season. 'My players had revenge in their minds after last year,' he said, referring to Arsenal's 2-0 defeat, which meant a top-four finish was out of their hands. But the Arsenal team coming to St James' Park this time around were a slightly more hardened group, and although it was Newcastle that started more brightly – a second-minute shot from Murphy hit the post and the Magpies were awarded a penalty that was later reviewed and the decision overturned – it was Arsenal that ultimately took all three points.

In fact, Newcastle fans were still effing and jeffing at the referee when Ødegaard was given too much space on the edge of the box and fired a left-foot drive past Pope to put the visitors ahead. Even the normally measured Howe was so incensed that Jason Tindall felt it necessary to extend a restraining arm to prevent him confronting Anthony Taylor, the fourth official, after the penalty 'decision'. It seemed that the Magpies had lost concentration at a crucial moment, allowing Arsenal to score with their first attack, and it was from that point on that the visitors seemed to take control away from the home side, showing how determined they were to fight Manchester City for the title. They won 2-0, a Schär own goal adding to Newcastle's misery.

Howe showed his frustration after the match:

> [It was] fine margins for us and we just came out on the wrong side of them. We missed some big chances in the game and it just wasn't quite there for us. I'm sure I'll look back at some moments and rue some moments we didn't get quite right. If Jacob's chance goes in early on, it's a totally different game. There

> are loads of things we'll look back on and think it could have gone our way and didn't. We have to take ownership of that. We're disappointed as I don't think we defended as well as we have done for the majority of the season. But we gave everything. It was a high-level game and two teams going right at each other.
>
> There were loads of chances there and we didn't put the ball in the net. We have done in our previous run of games. We didn't keep the ball well enough and were a bit loose in possession. When you give Arsenal transitions they're a very dangerous team and so it proved. The result will tell you they did [impose their style on the game], but in truth I think neither were dominant. It took that bit of quality to win it. It hinged on big moments.

It wasn't the start to the final month Howe and the team were looking for, and after feeling at home in third place during April, they slipped back down to fourth. It felt like they were on the brink of success but they couldn't afford to lose their grip on it, as so many times in the past getting over the finish line had been their downfall. It seemed like it would be a cruel and unnecessary twist in their fairy tale if things went wrong now. Howe was keen to make sure that everyone knew he believed in what the team were capable of. We all believed:

> We have four games remaining and need three results. Liverpool and other teams are coming. They are top level. We can only do what we can do and I believe in the character of the team to get it over the line.

The team and their character had another fight to overcome, an away game at Elland Road against Leeds, a team battling relegation. The match will henceforth be known as 'a tale of three penalties', as well as one that wobbled the normally unwobbly Howe. Leeds went ahead (boo!), then missed a golden opportunity from the penalty spot (yay!). Two minutes later Newcastle were awarded a spot kick of their own and scored, thanks to Wilson (yay again). They were then awarded another penalty when Junior Firpo handled inside his own area and Wilson did his magic yet again, putting the Magpies ahead (if you want to let out a whoop, let out a whoop).

That could have knocked the stuffing out of Leeds. However, they were down but not out, and with some resilience that they hadn't found for most of the season, they levelled the game (boo!) and it ended 2-2. It was a result that Howe couldn't quite make sense of when talking to BT Sport after the match:

> I'm struggling to make sense of it all. We started well. The first attack they get, they score. We hadn't created clear-cut chances. I thought we played well at times today without hitting our best form and we were rushed around the box. The character to come back is a huge positive. The way Wilson took his two penalties was outstanding. The second one is the most difficult, there are a lot of mind games and a lot of time to take the penalty.

With Wilson the man who saved the day for the team once again, there was another who upset the gaffer by storming over to him on the touchline. It happened in added time in the second half when the man was able to enter the

Newcastle technical area and push Howe before being escorted away by security. West Yorkshire Police issued a statement the following day:

> Police have charged a man with assault and entering the field of play following an incident at Elland Road football stadium during the Leeds United versus Newcastle United football match yesterday (13/5). The man has been bailed to appear before magistrates on July 21.

It was an incident that left Howe a little shaken once he'd had time to process what had happened:

> That was a real surprise. I was concentrating on the game. It was the last thing you think could happen. I can't repeat what he said but it makes you think 'what if?' It was personal to me. I can't remember if he pushed me or not, it was such a strange thing to happen. Moments like that make you think. We need to be mindful of security. Nobody should have to feel their personal safety is violated when trying to entertain the country. I didn't have time to be fearful, it was over in a flash. But it made me think about things after.

Three games to go and Newcastle welcomed the Seagulls to St James' Park on 18 May, with a fierce determination to take the points and provide more reassurance that they'd done enough to seal a place in the top four, where they'd sat for so long. That they were, as everybody had been saying for weeks now, heading to the Champions League. It was as if the team had heard a call to arms, and they went out on to the pitch with only one thing on their minds, handing out a thrashing. And that's what the Seagulls got. Being penned into their own half within minutes of the kick-off, Brighton looked like they were gasping for breath, and the game had only just started. The Seagulls had beaten Arsenal 3-0 the week before but were up against the force of the Magpies as Willock, Joelinton, Isak, Almirón and company forced their guests into a series of errors, rarely permitting them to hold on to the ball for more than a matter of seconds.

The match was as exciting as a game of football should be, full of relentless attack and physicality. Newcastle's first goal was an own goal, not the start to scoring any team wants but Newcastle took it. The second was a lot sweeter. Created by Trippier's free kick, the ball connected with big Dan Burn, who headed in beyond Brighton's keeper, Steele. St James' Park went ballistic. Burn stood like a giant in front of the home crowd, soaking in every moment. He'd scored his first Premier League goal for Newcastle, against the team he used to play for. Who'd have thought there was a time on the south coast when the defender could barely get a game for Brighton?

The second half saw the visitors come back with a goal but Newcastle weren't done scoring yet either, as Wilson scored his 18th goal of the season, meeting Almirón's pass and advancing 40 yards before side-footing home. Then Wilson held the ball up adroitly for Guimarães to apply an ecstatically received 12-yard finish. It really is a beautiful game, and Howe thought so too:

> I thought we were outstanding. I feel that's very much us at our best in that first half. We were relentless with what we did and full credit to the players for what they gave physically. That's how we

> want to play, fast and with high intensity. It was a brilliant performance, especially out of possession. But maintaining that sort of rhythm throughout is not easy and involves taking risks. When Brighton scored they made it a bit nervy. But we were mature with what we had to do during that period before we got the late goals. I thought we were fantastic in the details and the distances. We won the ball back so many times and we were just frustrated [in the first half] we hadn't scored from open play. We were reliant with set plays, but as first halves go, we were delighted by half-time. The players adapted really well and we were patient. The crowd helped us get over the line and the third goal was crucial.

The third goal, of course, was Wilson's, his 18th of the season, which meant that he was now Newcastle's highest scorer in a Premier League season since Shearer 19 years previously. Howe was full of praise for his striker:

> He's been incredible, and I feel that his performance was right up there with one of the best I've seen him play, purely from a tactical perspective. He kept going right until the end and his goalscoring record is excellent. I'm delighted for him, he's a huge player for us and a big presence in the dressing room.

My youngest son showed that he knows his stuff.

> Tommy: I think his goals are accurate, he doesn't necessarily power a shot, he thinks about where he wants to put the ball in the net. When Wilson has a free run I know he's going to score.

And Brighton boss Roberto De Zerbi was certain of one thing too: 'Newcastle deserve to qualify for the Champions League.'

And so to the question, what was needed now? It came down to a simple equation: Newcastle needed to win one of their remaining two games. They were four points clear of fifth-placed Liverpool with just two games to play, meaning they would finish in the top four if they could beat Leicester or Chelsea. Howe joked:

> I actually can't pronounce the CL words at the moment, they go funny against my lips. Nothing's been achieved. We're close but it's still so far away. We've tried not to talk about it in meetings. We can't take anything for granted.

However, when Liverpool could only manage a 1-1 draw at home to Villa, Newcastle were left needing just one point from those two matches to confirm their top-four finish.

> Henry: I was like Eddie, I didn't want to get my hopes up. I didn't want to believe until we were over the line. The Leicester game, we had beaten them 3-0 on Boxing Day so I knew we were ready. They had five players at the back, five defenders because they didn't want to be embarrassed. But we couldn't get a goal in, we had so many chances. But then they had a chance, in the 89th minute, they tapped it and Pope had to fall away, mid-height and save it. I wasn't worried until that moment Pope had to make a save as we were on top of them all match. I'm usually worried about watching. And I remember he said after the match, 'It's always nice to get involved,'

> which I thought was really funny because that was all his involvement as Newcastle had been trying to score all match.

Summoned up perfectly by my 11-year-old superfan, Henry articulated the resulting goalless draw that saw Newcastle United, the team that lots of pundits and football supporters would have placed money on being relegated the season before, now in the elite Champions League next season.

A tremendous atmosphere was generated by the home fans before kick-off. They waved their flags and, thanks to the amazing Wor Flags, a huge banner of Howe and the players was unfurled, emblazoned with the message: 'Bad times don't last but legends do.' It was in recognition of what Howe and the team had achieved, what they'd completed, what they'd done, not just as a football team for their supporters, but for the city as a collective, for the underdogs in every footballing community around the country, for the grassroots players who thought they knew about winning and losing, for the youngsters who thought that football had to be flash and fabulous and reminding them that it takes teamwork, hard work and the right man in charge to lead. When Howe took charge 19 months ago, Newcastle were 19th in the Premier League; courtesy of the point collected against Leicester, they'd finished in the top four.

They didn't need to do anything other than stumble over the line when it came to it. There was no need for a goal haul or fireworks to claim their glittering prize. It didn't need to be anything other than a clinical draw. But Newcastle didn't get that memo. They recorded 14 shots in the opening period, while Leicester barely ventured out of their own half, having just one touch in the opposition penalty box. Nick Pope was unemployed for about 90 minutes of the game. Wilson came within inches of adding to his tally, as did Miggy, Bruno and Isak. It was a shame that no one was able to break the deadlock in a match they completely dominated, having 78 per cent possession.

> Rob: I was at St James' Park. Everybody stayed behind, applauding and we were singing 'Que Sera, Sera, whatever will be will be, we're going to Wembley!' Then we'd sing, 'You'll never find a Mackem in Milan, we're off to Germany!' The songs were endless and everybody was congratulating each other, patting each other on the back like we, the 50,000 fans, had played the game ourselves. Everyone was patting backs and shaking hands and just constantly cheering. It went on for about half an hour, 45 minutes after the game. It was just electric. The sounds were deafening. The guy in front of me got very emotional and started to cry. I told him I remembered Newcastle being in the Champions League the first time round. I'd seen it before, I'd gone to Germany to watch a game. And now it was happening again.

Perhaps the scoreline wasn't as important as the matches that preceded it. Or rather the consistency of those games either side of the World Cup. A 17-match unbeaten run was, at one stage, the longest undefeated spell in any of Europe's top five leagues. Only Manchester City lost fewer Premier League matches all season. The Magpies showed a toughness others lacked, a reliability and a resolve that meant they could grind their way to securing a point, and their host of clean sheets in the first half of the season meant Nick Pope was hailed a hero in the same sentence as Miggy and Wilson, who both had inspiring scoring bursts at the beginning and near the end of the season.

This was Leicester's first clean sheet in six months but they had help in doing so – not only in their formation but that Newcastle weren't firing on all cylinders. Dean Smith, eager to plug his porous rearguard, played a 5-3-2 formation, with Harry Souttar as the extra centre-back. If visiting fans were happy with a draw, they were equally aggrieved that Bruno had seemingly got away with just a yellow card and should have been sent off for planting his studs on Soumaré's knee – VAR would have immediately agreed with the Foxes' supporters. But for now, this was all about the faithful Toon.

'It's a big relief, an amazing night to see the supporters react, it's incredible,' said Howe after the final whistle. But even ending a 20-year wait to return to the big stage, at the end of a campaign that also included a first major cup final appearance since 1999, didn't satisfy the Magpies' head coach. Not because he was arrogant, more that he was honest. He was someone who worked hard; this was just the way he was:

> Everyone will say, 'That's a great achievement.' All I can think of is that next challenge coming and then being prepared for that next challenge because you can't sit back and say, 'Right, I'm going to take a month off and go and relax on a beach.' It's the opposite, it's: 'Okay, how can we best now succeed in that next phase?' So it's very much you're always on a cycle of trying to improve. You're on sort of a conveyor belt that you can't get off.

The conveyor belt runs through the factory of which Howe and his team were site managers but had the support and backing of the factory owners, Staveley and Mehrdad Ghodoussi. Howe knew what a sense of unity fostered and shared among all levels of workers could bring to the team. Probably one of the reasons he asked the owners to come and chat to the squad before the end of the season:

> I invited Amanda and Mehrdad up to speak to the squad, I think it was ten days ago, roughly, just to have that contact with them, with the owners because it's so important as a club that we're one from top to bottom. They came in, they spoke to the players, they were absolutely brilliant. It was a nice moment, actually, just for everyone in the room to consolidate their thoughts on each other and then try to focus on the last few games that we had, and it made a positive impact on us.

It certainly had the desired effect. The players' smiles said it all as they stood clapping the crowd, hugging each other and their families as they savoured every moment of what they'd achieved over the past season. It was beyond a dream.

'I can't find the words, to be honest,' said Sean Longstaff, alongside Pope and Trippier in a post-match interview from the pitch, one that TV viewers would have to turn up the volume to hear because of the noise of the assembled crowd. 'If you told us two years ago this was going to happen, we wouldn't have believed you. We've beaten Juventus here 1-0 [in the Champions League], you see it on old DVDs. To be a part of this, I'm buzzing, to be fair.'

And so were the crowd. 'They've been unbelievable, the crowd,' said Pope, happy with yet another clean sheet. Tripps was equally praising and, as a player who had come into a relegation-threatened club that had now qualified for the Champions League, he knew what this success meant. 'We've shown great togetherness, we've earned the right to play in the Champions League. It will be incredible. The club has been through a tough moment, now they reap the rewards. We've worked so hard to be there next season, it means everything.'

> Alan: I was at St James' Park when Tino Asprilla scored a hat-trick against Barcelona 20-odd years ago. Watching them get there again brought back some good memories.

There were always going to be some camps that would suggest a top-four finish was the inevitable consequence of spending, which of course it couldn't have been. That's not to say it wouldn't and shouldn't be a plan for the future, but buying success can only happen when a club's expenditure dwarfs others. The provenance of Newcastle's funds might always remain a concern to some, while others see that moral and financial issues are entirely separate entities. But money wasn't the root of success here. It was the new owners who, showed they understood what running a football club looked like at every level. It was the talent. It was the fans. It was Howe.

You can debate nature versus nurture until you're a blue in the face but, ultimately, aren't we all guided by an example set by someone we admire? Gary Neville spoke at length about the benefits of having someone as down to earth, as stable and as principled as Howe leading the team:

> We've seen many different new owners come into clubs and appoint more fashionable managers, bought more

> fashionable players. I really like the players up at Newcastle, I like Eddie Howe, I like the work they've done and I hope they can maintain that humility as they try to progress into the Champions League. I hope they don't stray away from those principles and values they've got. It's really important they keep that. It suits the Newcastle community, the fans up there. They want a team they can rely upon.

Neville had certainly modified his stance since 2015 when many fans will remember him stating that Newcastle couldn't be a serious contender for players in the top league when it came up against the pull of London clubs. 'Does any top player now want to go and live in Newcastle?' he queried, before speculating that England's North East was 'being eased off football's map' and heading for 'irrelevance'.

But that was history and this was now, and at this very moment in time Newcastle had a manager who wanted more:

> I want success massively for this football club. The only difficult thing is that, although you feel like you've achieved something great, there is no trophy. We want to bring silverware here in the future. Our pre-season target? It certainly wasn't top four. We didn't feel that we were ready for that. After last season's battle with relegation it was whether we could consolidate and become a better team. To not have that flirtation with relegation, and try to give it a go. The lads have been unbelievable for me this year, I can't praise them enough. Their attitude, their mentality. It's just been incredible.

And so on to the thoughts of the summer, the new season, the pre-season training and, of course, the Champions League draw. There was also lots of talk, as there had been for months, about new summer signings and who'd be brought into the Newcastle fold. Signings had been wise so far, Newcastle had been sensible but equally willing to part with the money when needed. Over the past three transfer windows, £250m might sound a lot but consider their peers and the fact that Newcastle signed players when they desperately needed them. The threat of relegation prompted the first big buys but they'd only acquired who they needed and got value for money. In contrast, Manchester United had paid out more than that last summer alone, while Tottenham has spent similar over the past 18 months.

Newcastle could have made, and many suspect will make in the future, wild spending decisions. But so far it has been astute recruitment coupled with focused management of the players Howe inherited. Each purchased player, from the cheapest to the more expensive, has played their part, so you could argue that the strategy they're adopting at the moment is working. For example, in the win against Brighton that took Newcastle so close to a top-four finish, there was Trippier (£12m), Dan Burn (£12m) and Nick Pope (£10m), who, alongside Alisson of Liverpool, was the best goalie in the Premier League that season. You'd happily say you had three massive bargains there. Equally, Bruno Guimarães and Sven Botman, signings in the region of £35–£40m, are worth far more to the club than they cost, while the record fee of £63m went on Alexander Isak.

> Grampy: I didn't think he was worth it at the time but I can honestly say he's worth three times that

> amount now. When he came in initially I thought he was a stroppy sod, no good for the team and he wouldn't fit in. But then, we all know now, he's a world-class player. And he's really showing it, and he's still going to get better.

Although he was injured early on, Isak was a key player when it came to the second half of the season and the surge of victories. Having a top striker like Isak also meant Newcastle shouldn't be on the lookout for a striker the following season. It was all about promoting and pushing his potential. Then there was Anthony Gordon, who hadn't had a full season so had yet to prove his worth, although the signs were good, according to my father-in-law, who again was proven wrong by a signing.

> Grampy: I remember Gordon, the previous season when he played for Everton, made a bad tackle on Trippier, and Schär went over to sort out the problem. He was universally hated at that point by Newcastle fans and I thought, when he was signed, that he would bring his attitude to Newcastle and he'd be a waste of money. But his attitude is spot on. Completely different to what I thought, which was that he would be a stroppy, horrible player – a bit like I thought about Isak – but he's the complete opposite. He's one of our top players. Even when he got cross with Howe, he was out of order by not being happy about going off but he apologised afterwards and he said he was wrong and that Howe was right, and you see the player now, he's unbelievably good. And he has a great attitude. Definitely money well spent.

Arguably, though, Newcastle paid over the odds for Chris Wood in January 2022, as he scored just four Premier League goals in 35 appearances. They did, however, do well to recoup much of that £25m fee a year later when he went to Nottingham Forest. The less said about the hat-trick he scored against Newcastle in the 2023 Boxing Day match the better, eh? The point is that what has been spent so far doesn't seem frivolous or wasted.

But summer 2023 was fast approaching and the new season was going to be Newcastle's most important yet, and they were playing with the big boys now. We know there's a willingness to spend but always within the parameters of the Premier League and UEFA's respective FFP regulations. Of course, we know they can deviate from their plan when necessary. A £40m outlay on Anthony Gordon, for example, was beyond their intended January spend, as was the club-record fee for Alexander Isak in the summer. But that has also led to a growing revenue, which is relative to the self-proclaimed 'big six' clubs. Tottenham, for example, had a turnover of nearly £450 million in 2021/22, which was more than double Newcastle's. And don't get me started on Manchester City the monetary figures for that blew my mind upon researching and I needed to sit down. But for the Magpies, where there's a will, there's a way, and the hope now was that increased pricing and commercial attractiveness would result from the potential winning of trophies and playing European football. Increased revenue and success on the pitch go together like pie and chips.

Chapter 13

You're Only as Good as Your Last Game

'The pain you feel now is motivation for tomorrow.'

Eddie Howe

SO THE Magpies had risen. It would be fair to say that this would be a natural point for the story to end as the focus on 2022/23 has taken up the bulk of the pages. The beginning, the middle and the end of such a tale is complete but, let's be honest, who doesn't enjoy the 'what happened next' chapter that comes after you've finished the main event. So here you go. The rising of this magnificent team has been charted, so now it's time for them to soar.

There has always been a consistent message from Howe when it comes to signings and spending, and that boils down to him wanting to invest shrewdly. Overspending wasn't an option, as he made clear before the summer:

> Unfortunately, players don't come cheap, especially good players. Yes, we're going to have to spend a certain amount of money. How much that is, I don't

> know. I still don't know what my budget is at this moment in time, but there will have to be some expenditure. It will have to be controlled. It will have to be under FFP restrictions, which we've worked under and will continue to work under. They're definitely impacting us and what we'll be able to do.

But when you've achieved the success Newcastle have in such a short space of time, spending 'big' was probably one of their only options, especially if they wanted to match their success season after season. But, equally, if they only wanted to focus on the season in front of them, competing in the Champions League was going to be tough if they didn't have the squad to match the pressure.

> I think we've massively overachieved this year for where we were at the start of the season, and to keep overachieving – and that's what we're going to have to do to match the expectation – is going to be our biggest challenge. I don't know if it's something you look forward to, but the dynamic will have changed for us.

For fans, a marquee signing might very well be a player to thrill and entertain or to provide hope for the future. Often the price of a player reflects the quality being purchased but it could just be the value that the buying and selling clubs are willing to agree on. Asked whether his wish list would include marquee signings, Howe said:

> Yes, there would be players we'd love to bring in that would be classified in that bracket, I'm sure. For me, it's more about the role they can fulfil in the team

> – whether that's viewed positively or as a marquee signing, then great. I'm not in my mind thinking, *We have to have one of those players that ticks that box for the supporters.* As much as I'd love to do that, it's about finding the right player in the right position who I think makes us better.

Back in 2017 there was a similar issue about Newcastle needing to spend on marquee players but for totally different reasons. The late Freddy Shepherd was keen for Ashley to spend in the summer as he wasn't sure the current squad were fit for the Premier League. The former owner knew that Rafa Benítez had a hard job on his hands getting in the big players that were so desperately needed. In one of his last interviews with *The Chronicle*, Shepherd said:

> You are competing against people with a bottomless pit where money is concerned. It's very simple. I think he needs somebody who will make the town buzz. Signing Shearer was big news. We'd been working on it a long time.

Times like that seem a distant memory now but still sit within many fans' concerns about buying the right players. It was a case of looking around the world, according to Howe. Finding the right 'depth' of players being the main objective:

> When you're sat in my shoes, it's [the budget] never as big as you want it to be. It's a difficult one because we go into a lot of competitions next year, so we need the depth. I think this year we've been light, certainly in certain areas of the pitch. We've carried – in the

> second half of the season – four midfielders. You're one injury away from a very difficult situation so I think we need a little bit more depth. We're not there yet, but we're suffering from injuries. Certainly that's a concern for us in that we do need to bolster our resources. We can't be looking at one or two injuries and we're in a difficult position.

So, in the first signing of the summer, confirmed just before the squad flew off to the US for the Premier League Summer Series, please give a very warm welcome to Italian international and AC Milan player Sandro Tonali. The 23-year-old arrived on a five-year contract for £55m, making him the most expensive Italian footballer of all time, but the star just wanted to play the beautiful game:

> I want to repay the trust on the pitch, giving it my all, as I always have. I'm really excited about playing at St James' Park, I can't wait to feel the warmth of the fans.

The Italian didn't feature heavily on initial lists of potential targets being touted, but Newcastle were encouraged to instigate the deal when they realised he was available within their budget and would offer both flexibility and a top level of athleticism. While talk in the previous few months had been on trying to sign a specialist holding midfielder, Tonali would offer a far more dynamic style to the position. Howe was pleased:

> He's an exceptional talent and has the mentality, physicality and technical attributes to be a great fit for us. At 23, Sandro already has important experience as

> a key player in one of Europe's top leagues and in the Champions League, as well as playing for his country. But he also has the opportunity and potential to grow and evolve with us, and I'm excited to add him to our squad as we approach the exciting season ahead.
>
> Sandro is one of those players who can elevate everyone around him. He'll fit in really well to how we play. Marquee is not necessarily the right word. For me it's good players and bringing in players who will elevate the group. The early signs are very positive. He's a great lad as well, so he has fitted in really well so far. I can't wait to see him in a Newcastle shirt.

It was a good start. Trippier, among others, tried to make him feel welcome, and when Tonali came to the training ground the first time he made sure that the Italian knew he was speaking from his own experience of joining a club in a different country. 'If you need any help, I'm always here. Just to help you settle. I know how hard it is to move to a different country so I'm here if you need any help, about the city, the team, or anything, I'm here. I want to make you feel welcome,' Tripps told him.

But there was talk among many fans that Tonali may not have been keen on leaving AC Milan, a club also in Champions League and in a city that didn't have the wet, windy, north-eastern UK weather conditions that Tyneside had.

> Rob: Like most Newcastle fans I was very surprised to sign such a big Italian player, especially Tonali, as he's a massive Milan fan and probably didn't want to leave.

And the feeling that perhaps the Italian wasn't quite so keen on the blustery north of England wasn't helped by the fact he spent just 24 hours in Newcastle before heading off on holiday. So it was a shrewd move from the Italian to then post on his Instagram account a video that documented his first few days at the club, with the soundtrack to his clip of 'Getting Started' by Sam Fender, a high-profile supporter of Newcastle.

Anthony Gordon was keen to get to work with his new team-mate and to be playing with 'one of the best midfielders in the world':

> I knew him from his early days at Brescia. I remember seeing some clips of him before he went to Milan. He has excelled and is one of the top midfielders in the world. It shows the direction we're going in. I'm really looking forward to playing with him.

And Dan Burn was equally excited about what buying a player like Tonali signalled to the footballing world:

> It's like a mentality coming. It's some statement when you think we're bringing in someone who played for AC Milan in the Champions League last season and he's stepping into a team built from players who've grown with the club. A couple of years ago we couldn't have dreamed of a signing like him. He's a sign of where we are and what we want to become.

Others agreed:

> Terry: I liked the look of him, for sure. We were spending money in the right way again and I liked

> the fact he was an international player, he was young but he obviously knew what he was doing. Hopefully he'll be able to play both deep and more advanced in the park and help Bruno at those crucial moments.
>
> Sharon: I'll be honest, I thought he was a great signing.

Howe was keen to dispel rumours that his new signing didn't want to come to Tyneside, and when he made his debut against Rangers, on the pitch for 45 minutes as part of their pre-season training, the manager chose to address fans' concerns:

> Sandro is very, very proud to be here, and proud to wear the shirt and represent the club. That was made very clear to me very early, otherwise we wouldn't have committed to the transfer. We don't have any kind of desire to drag anyone to Newcastle – they have to want to run there with no shoes on. That's the mentality we want because you have to have that togetherness, spirit and desire to do well. That can only come from a desire to play for the club.

Tonali made a great impression as he completed 45 minutes at Ibrox on 19 July. Howe was equally praising of his talent on the pitch:

> I was very impressed with Sandro. I thought he was excellent. Everything we hoped he would bring, he did in that first 45 minutes. He was very calm and composed, and technically he was at a very high level. He built good relationships with the players around

> him, and looked at home in a black-and-white shirt. It was a great start for him.
>
> We had a quick nod and a smile after the game. I think you could see he was enjoying himself by his body language and how he plays. He looked like he was enjoying himself, certainly with some of the players around him, in that first half. I'd be surprised if he didn't enjoy playing that type of football, with the players that he's with. There was a really attractive style. I thought we moved the ball really well, and he was pivotal to that.

After the Rangers game, Newcastle flew from Glasgow to the US as part of their Premier League Summer Series that saw them and five other clubs take part in some competitive matches in a different environment ahead of the new 2023/24 campaign. With a huge fanbase out in the States, the team were treated very much to the same love and support that they find on Tyneside, Elliot Anderson in particular paying tribute to the level of Geordie support:

> Everywhere we went, in all three cities, the number of black-and-white shirts we saw was phenomenal.

Training and competing in Atlanta, Philadelphia and New Jersey was an experience the youngster and the rest of the squad would never forget, a chance for some team bonding – especially for the new players, as Dan Burn said of his new team-mate:

> He's quiet, really quiet. I can't tell you what he's like, not yet. I'm just being honest with you; we haven't spent enough time together. You don't just step into

> a team like ours. I'm not saying we're amazing or anything, but we're very specific in what's needed and what the manager wants from you. It takes time to learn.

It should also be noted that the Italian star was probably more on the quiet side while he got to grips with the English language. Shay Given, who was working as a club ambassador in the US when the team went over, enjoyed meeting the new signing and was impressed by his grasp of the English language:

> I had a bit of lunch with Sandro and Tripps and a few others and just asked him about his English. I'm not saying it was brilliant, but I was surprised with how good it was; I'm not sure how proficient my Italian would be after a couple of weeks over there. He's having a couple of lessons here but he told me that once he gets back home to Tyneside it'll be lessons every day. He strikes me as a very intelligent guy. He's certainly a very intelligent footballer.

While Miggy is 'always smiling', according to Howe, Tonali is a bit more like the boss when it comes to showing emotions, another good reason the US tour was a good bonding experience for everyone:

> From what I've seen of Sandro and what I know of him, he's happy inside. People probably accused me of something similar – I can guarantee I'm happy but sometimes I don't show it. He's been really, really good. He greets me with a smile every morning and he's built some good friendships already. I've got no

> concerns about his happiness. This trip will really help him settle in with the group. You get to spend all your free time with your team-mates; there's no better way to get to know them and feel acclimatised to the team than actually spending time with them. And the same goes on the pitch, so, when you play a game, suddenly the dynamic of you and your team-mates changes. This is all an important part of his process in learning how to play for Newcastle.

Tripps was keen to protect the new player when it came to media scrutiny and fitting in, and he wasn't worried that he hadn't seen a different side to Tonali, away from the quietness:

> It's early days. Sandro speaks for himself as a player. I've played against him a few times for Atlético and for England and we've bought a top-quality player who can help move us forward. Behind the scenes, he interacts. He's not been here long and his English is getting better, but it'll take him a bit of time. On the pitch, his football does the talking.

It was a sentiment that Shay Given shared when he looked on in the US – a quiet personality who spoke volumes on the pitch. In fact, with a football, Tonali was as loud as they come:

> Just watching him in training over here, he makes the game look so easy – he's a yard ahead of people in his head. He sees things other people don't see. He's pure quality.

My husband clearly agreed.

> Chris: I thought he seemed a bit nervy at first, but then he started blending in and played really well. Of course, then it all went a bit wrong and the gambling stuff came out …
>
> [More on that later, of course.]

What is pertinent to say at this point is that Tonali was a hit with the fans the moment he stepped foot in Tyneside. At the beginning of July, fresh from a flight from Milan, he went to look at a house and was stopped by passing fans. The young player was more than happy to pose for photos, realising early on that the supporters were some of the greatest in the world.

They, in turn, weren't disappointed with their new player. In his Premier League debut against Aston Villa on 12 August he scored Newcastle's first goal of the season after just six minutes. 'Build this man a statue' came the comments online. It was up there with Isak's debut but, for many, seeing such a seasoned player in their black-and-white shirt proved Tonali was the real deal. The crowd at St James' Park went wild. It was a dream start for the team in general, getting off to a 5-1 win against Aston Villa, with Isak netting two goals and Wilson and Barnes also scoring. I do wonder whether Unai Emery would have thought to himself at this point, *What if?*

Howe said after the match:

> Sandro was magnificent. It was a tight, tough game decided by our ruthlessness, and we can improve. But we want our supporters to dream.

The last point was in reference to the 50,000-strong singing of 'we're going to win the league'.

> Henry: I loved him, lots of people did. He was so passionate. I loved the fact that you could hear the new chant the Toon Army had made for him.

Ahh, yes, the chant. To the tune of Los Lobos's cult classic 'La Bamba', the lyrics are pretty colourful:

> *Sandro Tonali, Sandro Tonali,*
> *He drinks Moretti and eats spaghetti,*
> *He hates f****** Sunderland.*

Now a bit of a memory, too, of course, but not for long – at the time of writing there was still hope that Tonali would be back in action for the start of the 2024/25 season.

Newcastle's second signing of the summer, Harvey Barnes, who cost £38m, had this to say:

> Newcastle is such an ambitious club and Sandro shows that ambition. He shows they're not happy with where they finished last year, they want to keep improving. It shows the direction the club wants to go in. That was a big reason I was so determined to come here. And he looks great on the ball. If you're making the runs, he'll get you in. He'll be a joy to play with.

Barnes, 25, had been courted by Tottenham, Aston Villa and West Ham before the summer transfer market officially opened, but when Newcastle made a play for the winger, the decision was black and white for the former Leicester City player:

> I'm delighted. It's an amazing club and, for me, it's a massive opportunity to be involved in a successful team that's doing exciting things, so I'm absolutely buzzing to be here.
>
> I think it's an attacker's dream to come into a team like this; it's high-paced, it's physically demanding but you can see the reward of that with the chances created and goals scored. I certainly think I'll suit Newcastle's style.

Howe seemed equally delighted to sign a wide forward who was set to replace Saint-Maximin, a player leaving Tyneside for Saudi Arabian club Al-Ahli:

> Harvey is an exciting talent who I've admired for a long time, so I'm delighted to welcome him to Newcastle. He's strong, quick and very good technically, and he showed last season, in particular, that he has an eye for goal from wide positions.

I asked my sons what it's like when you lose a player.

> Tommy: Sometimes it makes me feel a bit annoyed because when Chris Wood joined Nottingham Forest, we played them and he scored a hat-trick against us and I was like, 'Why couldn't he do that for our team?' It made me cross. I do feel sad, though. Some players can be really good at football and then we lose them and we're less good.

> Henry: Of course it's sad, Mum, 'cos they're people that you've supported. [Shrugs.] With Maxi it was hard because he'd been with us for a long time. But

> the club is the club, that's what you have to remember. You follow the club, not the player.

Ahh, wise words from a youngster to a sentimental old bird like myself. But I get it. In a leaving statement from Saint-Maximin, he too showed emotion when he wrote to fans in a social media post:

> I fell for Newcastle, I had great opportunities to leave during dark days, but that was too late I was already in love, I wanted, I needed, I had to stay for helping my team to save the club from Premier League relegation because it meant the world for me. Of course, during those dark days some may have had their doubts, but I always believed in this club and look where we are today, it's just so beautiful. I'm leaving Newcastle as it should always have been and that's my greatest trophy because I was a part of it. Even though this chapter has ended, the story never stops. Newcastle is home now. I'll continue to be your biggest supporter.

Maxi, it's been a pleasure.

Talking of pleasure, there was a young player who went with the team on their pre-season jaunt to the States who was causing quite a stir. Every so often, one or two of the most promising talents in Newcastle's academy are invited to train with the first-team squad as a snippet of experience for what being a top-class footballer entails.

Lewis Miley was only 16 and a few weeks out of school when he received the summons from Howe in 2022, and from that point on there was no looking back, as Howe explained:

> The biggest compliment I can give Lewis is that, straightaway, he looked like part of the group. For someone so young to survive, technically, within the first-team group is no mean feat. Some of the drills we do are very difficult. Lewis survived in those drills; that's a very big thing.

Miley had been part of the academy since the age of seven and was invited to Saudi Arabia in December last year with the first team for their warm-weather training. To give you some context, Anthony Gordon said it took him several months to get to grips with Howe's training instructions, finding that he 'couldn't always understand' the complex tactical instructions given to him.

So it was that Miley joined the squad in Atlanta in July and the now 17-year-old held his own among the big boys. Howe was impressed with what he saw when Miley played against Chelsea on 26 July:

> That was a very mature performance tonight against high-class opposition and will do him the world of good. He's shown he can play in front of a crowd, which is not always a given. I'm delighted for him.

He had, of course, come up against Chelsea before, having made his Premier League debut against them in the last game of the season on 28 May when he came on in the 76th minute. It made him Newcastle's youngest-ever Premier League player. But the decision after that about whether to keep him in the bosom of the Magpies squad rather than loan him out was apparently unanimous – he was 'some boy' and they wanted him in the first-team pool. The only point up for debate at that point seemed to be whether the

6ft 2in teenage prodigy had started using a razor or not. Howe outlined his plans for the teenager:

> The plan has been consistent in my mind. He'll stay with us this season. There's no thought of sending him on loan. For me he's too young to be exposed to that at the moment. I think he needs to stay with his family and to train with us and to learn and develop around the players we have. I don't think he's surprised me because I've seen it for six months, including at the back end of last season, just how well he was developing and how strong he looked in the group.
>
> Physically is always the biggest test for someone so young but you've seen him today – he's a very, very good athlete, he's strong and a good size and he looks like he can handle the environment he's in. The next step is to push him and develop him and I'm sure he'll get minutes this year. The biggest challenge for Lewis will be to handle the attention and exposure. It's dealing with that and then waiting for his opportunity while keeping his head. He'll have a lot of people in his ear. All those things contribute to how you handle success, and when it comes early that can be difficult. We'll try and guide him and educate him as best we can.

Miley went on to feature in every pre-season fixture in the US, playing so naturally and gracefully with Tonali and others that he looked like he'd been playing with the team for years. 'The future will be the judge for Lewis but he's had an early taste of high-level football and taken everything in his stride,' said Howe.

Miley grew up as one of four brothers in the small County Durham hill town of Stanley, and as a pupil at Tanfield School honed his close control and first-touch skills playing in his year group's local title-winning futsal team. Howe said of him:

> For someone so young he's got a good perspective on life and sport. He's very calm, very polite, very respectful. But he's also keen to show his qualities. The difficult decision we've had is that he's so young and you want to protect him and not expose him too soon, which can have a negative effect. But he's looked ready to be around us and be involved and train with us and he has for some time now.

And my son has certainly taken a shine to him.

> Henry: Lewis is one of my favourite players; he doesn't give up. I remember in a Sunderland match, he had a horrible tackle against him but he got straight back up, wiped the mud off his face and carried on like a true Geordie. It's quite unusual in football to see that, but I loved it.

To finish off their pre-season preparations, Newcastle welcomed Villarreal to St James' Park at the beginning of August, and watching in the stands was a third new signing of the summer, Southampton defender Tino Livramento. In a deal worth an initial £32m, the 20-year-old signed a five-year contract with the club and Howe was, as ever, most pleased with his new full-back:

> Tino is a very talented young player with an exciting future ahead of him so we're delighted to sign him. At 20, he already has lots of attributes that I admire, but he also has the potential and drive to really grow with this team. I'm looking forward to working with him and to seeing him develop in a Newcastle shirt.

The young Englishman was eager to show his appreciation for the club and for his new boss too, but, more importantly, to get the chance to play football after suffering with an injury for most of the previous season that saw him appear only twice for Southampton:

> The way the manager plays football is really attractive and I feel like it suits me as a player. With how well the team did last season, the trajectory that we're on now, I'm just looking forward to being a part of that. To be able to learn from Kieran Trippier is another big thing for me. Hopefully he teaches me how to become a better player and a better full-back.

It was, many fans and pundits considered, quite a shrewd move. To develop a young full-back under the guidance of Tripps, who at 32 would probably find playing all the games the team would face domestically and in the Champions League quite tough. Well, of course, no one is ousting Tripps from his position, but it was good to know that there was potential for Livramento, in the years to come, to eventually take over. He still wasn't a well-enough known signing for others, though.

> Chris: He was a bit under the radar for me, to be honest; there were other names that were being

> touted around that seemed bigger and more exciting. Although I remember Dad talking about him a lot and saying he liked the sound of him. But then, I'm probably the wrong person to ask. I was expecting Newcastle, bear in mind they're about to play Champions League football for the first time in 20-odd years, to buy in the likes of Ronaldo and Gareth Bale.

The start of the Premier League, as mentioned above for Tonali's debut, couldn't have gone better for the Magpies. A 5-1 victory over Aston Villa was, however, a bit of a flash in the pan as they went on to lose their next three games – against Manchester City, Liverpool and Brighton & Hove Albion. Despite the latter of the three being a 'thumping' away loss, 3-1, Howe wasn't worried:

> You can lose any game in the Premier League – we've lost three in a row and we have to take responsibility. Man City game was tight, although we weren't great; Liverpool we were excellent for a half and should have won; and today hinged on moments. It's important I don't overreact, and the support meant so much. It's never lost on me how difficult the Premier League is – it's ruthless. If you sway your focus, you have big problems. Our focus hasn't been swayed ... determined to be successful in the league. But we know the demands placed upon us will be extreme. This is a warning that we can't be swayed in such a tough league.

Brighton fans were quick to compound the Magpies' losing streak with chants of 'Champions League, you're having a laugh' echoing from the stands. But no one takes heed of such goading, and Newcastle had just had their group stage announced, with their first game on 19 September, away against AC Milan.

A bit of a boost came in the Premier League three days before the Milan trip with a 1-0 victory over Brentford. It was enough, perhaps, to refocus the team on their capabilities as they entered their first Champions League match with their heads held high. They came away from Italy with an impressive 0-0 draw. To play last season's semi-finalists in their first game of the campaign could have been daunting, the expectation heavy on their shoulders. But they showed grit.

> Chris: To go away to a team like AC Milan, I thought it would be a tough, tough game, so to come away with a draw was a fantastic start to our campaign. We played well, we could have won and that was really pleasing to see.

But others felt that Newcastle looked like they were struggling from the word go, with pundits describing their 'limp performance' as 'underwhelming'.

'If they want to emerge from the toughest of the eight Champions League groups, Newcastle will have to show more than they mustered in Milan,' said a Sky Sports journalist.

'I think they got away with a draw thanks to some almighty saves by Pope,' said fan Craig. 'He was top of his game, thank goodness, and I think knocked out eight shots from Milan to keep a clean sheet!'

> Steve: We only had one shot at goal, with Longstaff in injury time. We didn't look like we were fighting,

> we were just counting down the minutes to get the draw and I know we can do much better.

But Tonali, Milan's former player, wasn't disappointed with the performance against his old team:

> It was emotional. We take this draw and point, a point we fought to get and we're happy about.

Howe insisted the point Newcastle took back to Tyneside would 'look better as time goes on'. So was it nerves, Eddie?

> You can't underestimate the difficulties of coming here. The emotion of the game, new experiences – we had to take a lot on board today. I thought the crowd were very good for Milan. It was a hostile atmosphere and the players had to adjust to that, and that's why I don't think you can underestimate the performance and point. It will look better and better as time goes on. There were new experiences for a lot of us tonight and hopefully we can grow from this.

Man-of-the-match Pope was equally happy with the situation, in an 'I'm-pleased-that's-over-with' kind of way:

> I'm proud of the performance tonight. If you can keep it to a zero you have a good chance. I was kept busy but the boys did a great job to help me out too.

Tripps said in the post-match interview:

> I'm feeling very positive. The whole team, the lads that came on and the lads that travelled gave a great

> account of ourselves. Certain moments we could have done a bit better. Everyone put their bodies on their line, we've come a long way, we deserve to be in the Champions League, we have a right to be here.

And that was the point, wasn't it? They'd earned the right to be playing AC Milan and, no matter what was going to happen over the next few months, that should never be forgotten. We know, of course, how the Champions League campaign ended. It wasn't the fairy tale ending that we all hoped for but, again, hope is a strange phenomenon. You hope Newcastle will win, and in their very next Premier League match they did, 8-0 against Sheffield United. What a match that was. Goals for Longstaff, Burn, Botman, Wilson, Gordon, Almirón, Guimarães and Isak. Then three days later a win against Manchester City in the third round of the Carabao Cup – and a first competitive start for Lewis Miley.

But as victories go, I think it's important that one more big one gets mentioned. Newcastle's second game in the Champions League group stage against PSG.

St James' Park welcomed the French giants to the stadium in true Geordie style, making sure it would be a Wednesday night no one would ever forget. And it wasn't. You wouldn't have been able to sleep through the noise the Chapel on the Hill made that evening. It was deafening, even by their standards.

> Steve: I've never seen a fanbase at 0-0 celebrating tackles in their own half. Honestly, incredible atmosphere.

With a result that saw them go top of their Champions League group, the mighty Toon won 4-1 against the losing finalists of the previous season. It was an unbelievable night for those there, those watching at home or in pubs and clubs around the country, or around the world. Little ol' St James' Park roaring its team into the lead as the Magpies scored on 20 minutes, thanks to Almirón converting an Isak rebound. The crowd roared louder still when the second goal came from boyhood superfan big Dan Burn, who powered his header over the line but had to wait a few minutes before VAR could confirm there was no offside or handball. It was worth the wait.

And there was still more to come. If PSG wanted a break from the relentless goals being scored against them or the relentless rain beating down on them, they were going to get neither. Straight after half-time there was another homegrown talent waiting for his big moment in the shape of Sean Longstaff, who scored the third goal. The same Longstaff who admitted that he wanted Mbappé's shirt after the game 'for his little brother'. I'd wager that there would have been more youngsters after his own shirt when the final whistle blew. If you weren't watching, you might not have believed what happened. You might have had to pinch yourself. You might have been drunk – Longstaff put money on that his family probably were:

> My family will be proud, they'll be drunk as well! They don't go out on a Wednesday night but they might now. It's some night. I think we knew as a group it would be special with the atmosphere. But for me and Dan Burn to score tonight is surreal, I'm lost for words! There are a few who thought three years ago they were out the door. Since the takeover

> it has been amazing. It's been an unbelievable night and I'm over the moon. This is the elite of the elite and they've got some of the best players in the world. To go against them was amazing. There's still stuff to improve on, but tonight we'll celebrate.

PSG came back with a goal of their own in the 56th minute but it was Schär who decided that Newcastle needed the last word, with a goal in the 91st minute, sealing not just a win, but a triumphant victory over one of the best in the world. Kylian Mbappé and his team-mates looked shell-shocked by the sodden occasion, overrun by the black-and-white shirts and a home crowd that were cheering every tackle their heroes made.

Newcastle were without several key figures too: Sven Botman, Callum Wilson and Joelinton were among the injured. But it didn't matter. They had something more than PSG would ever have, that unwavering, unyielding, relentless home-crowd support, as a smiling Howe appreciated:

> What the supporters gave us tonight was incredible. They're such a good team. We had to defend really well, and we did. I thought, collectively, our spirit and our energy was excellent. We created the positive things we had in the first half from really aggressive pressing, everything that's a hallmark of ours when we play well. Then, second half we had to dig deep and get over the line.

Rewatching the game the next day, the following week and then almost six months later still gives me the same goosebumps it did when I watched it at the time. But I probably find it more incredible that the wider footballing world, those who aren't part of the Toon Army or living in Tyneside or have any affiliation with the club – most of them have their own allegiances – loved watching that match. It was like Newcastle had become a team that the collective wanted to root for.

'I'm a Manchester United fan,' said one, 'and I lived in Sunderland for a few years. But I'm delighted to see Newcastle beat PSG 4-1 at home in the Champions League. Congratulations to the Geordie nation, your fans are a credit to your football club.'

'I'm a Wednesday fan,' said another, 'but was yelling my head off when that Schär goal went in. Brilliant game, congrats to the Geordies.'

'Standing ovation from an Arsenal fan here. Brilliant play from the Toon, and that last goal was amazing!'

'Chelsea fan here. I was in a bar in Tenerife full of English fans from all different clubs. Each goal that went in, the bar was rocking. Unbelievable.'

Howe talked up his team's 'spirit and energy' afterwards but it was hard for him to do justice to what he'd witnessed. 'There are so many stories to talk about,' he said. And it goes without saying that the fans will revel in those stories for years to come. Certainly in the Burn and Longstaff household at every family gathering.

But sadly, the Champions League campaign was over before it really began. The highs and the lows of the club going hand in hand. They'd qualified for the Champions League for the first time since 2002/03 but suffered multiple injury problems during the season and could only name seven subs to Milan's 11.

> Chris: Injuries ... Injuries played a major part. Suddenly you're playing all these extra games as well

> as Premier League games and you don't have the pool of players to use. I'm gutted for them.

Howe said:

> We've learned a lot. We went into this season knowing the power of the squad and how important that would be, but unfortunately we lost that power and ultimately we went into Champions League games with very few options.
>
> I feel for the players. I've seen what they've given and how committed they've been. I can't fault them at all. It's painful for me and for them because I know how professional they are and how they want to achieve success. Any time you don't achieve what you want and have a setback and disappointment you have to use it as fuel. That has always been my way. The pain you feel now is motivation for tomorrow and now we have to focus on the Premier League. For me there's nothing but positive thoughts about the team and what they're giving, but now we have to make sure we're consistent in the Premier League. I'm desperately disappointed. It's tough to take.

Another tough bit of news to take was that of Tonali's future with the club. In October 2023 Italy's football federation banned him from playing football for ten months for breaking the country's gambling regulations and ordered that the midfielder must spend the following eight months on a rehabilitation programme.

Newcastle said that Tonali would participate in 'a therapeutic plan and educational programme in Italy consisting of 16 commitments', and Howe was keen to stress that the club had no knowledge of any potential betting breaches when they signed him:

> You make a decision at the time with the knowledge you have. We really liked him as a footballer and had no idea that this was even a possibility. There's a frustration and a disappointment that we're not going to have a quality player for a period of time. It shows nobody knows what tomorrow will bring. It's a valuable lesson. We need a squad robust enough to deal with these things. It's part of life and football.

Speaking about Tonali's mindset, Howe said:

> From the moment this happened, his training performances have been very good. His mood is the same. It's there in the background and I'm sure these are difficult times for him.

Howe's supportive stance has been welcomed by The Big Step, a campaign group lobbying to end all gambling advertising and sponsorship in football. It forms part of Gambling with Lives, a charity established by those bereaved by betting-related suicides.

'Footballers are human and if they are suffering from addiction they deserve empathy and support, not lengthy bans,' The Big Step said in a statement. 'Every football game is wall-to-wall with gambling ads, not just across shirts but around stadiums and related media content.'

Tonali admitted that he'd placed 40 to 50 bets on football between August and October in 2023, including four bets on Newcastle to win. While Tonali played in four matches that he'd bet on, the FA were satisfied that the integrity of the game was not called into question:

> While Tonali did place bets on his own team, all of those bets were for his team to win the match in question. Tonali's betting pattern is consistent in this regard and there has been no damage to integrity or perception of the integrity of the game as a whole.

At the time of writing, Tonali is set to return to competitive football for the start of the 2024/25 season provided there are no further breaches.

> Henry can't wait: Everyone deserves a second chance, we all make mistakes, Mum.

* * *

What's the future for Newcastle then? With a manager who spent admirable time shadowing Atlético Madrid's Diego Simeone and Rayo Vallecano's Andoni Iraola (now ironically in charge of his previous team), during a post-Bournemouth sabbatical, Howe has shown he's a character who wants to learn, wants to know his players and wants to invest in every area of their development.

Could another manager have spotted that Joelinton was more of a masterful midfielder than a flop of a £40m centre-forward? Would another coach have ignored constant chat that Fabian Schär could only operate in a Premier League back three and then reinvented the Switzerland international as an outstanding centre-half in a back four? Could anyone other than Howe and his team have made Miggy a goal threat?

The PIF money has helped, undoubtedly, but the accolade of Champions League qualification at the end of a season originally intended to be all about finishing in the top half of the table is principally down to Howe confounding the doubters. Confounding the believers too. His amalgamation of emotionally sound management and thorough coaching that requires high standards means that the Magpies have been transformed under his care. Elevated from relegation dodgers to Champions League returners within a year. They play high-energy, crowd-pleasing football. They have players that want to do the best for the man in charge, for the team, for the fans. They have a fanbase that not only believes in the players but believes in the whole club again. They've silenced the London-based analysts who said that such a club would be 'unbuyable' because it was 'too far north' of the capital.

> Steve: You'll be hard-pressed to find anyone criticising the Saudis up Tyneside. We have a lot of faith in them because they have a lot of faith in us as a city and as a club. We were dismissed for so long during Ashley's ownership, it was like people forgot we existed as anything other than a bit-part player in a London boys' league. We're a worldwide force to be reckoned with!

After finishing in the top four in 2022/23, last season wasn't so inspiring. The Magpies were knocked out of the FA Cup in the sixth round, they dropped out of the Champions League after the group stage, they were knocked out of the Carabao Cup in the fifth round and they finished seventh in the Premier League. We'd love to report that they finished the season with a spot in European football, but Manchester United beating Manchester City in the FA Cup Final meant the Magpies were out of Europe altogether.

And in July 2024, Amanda and her husband Mehrdad decided that their time in Newcastle had come to an end. Amanda said she was 'devasted' to be leaving the club:

> We did a great job and it has been a privilege to be part of it. I didn't want to get in Newcastle's way, it's got to be about what's best for Newcastle. Mehrdad and I are keen to be hands-on. We're hard-working people and I love football.

Meanwhile, my husband and sons are optimistic for the future.

> Chris: I'm sad to see them go but I guess it means that they think they've done their job, they've given Newcastle a base from which to fly and become a massive club. We won't forget what they've done for us.

> Henry (after the FA Cup Final): I wonder what might have been. But Dad told me that it doesn't matter because, when you follow a team like Newcastle, you're always chasing the dream. And I've seen that dream come true once before. I'm sure to see it again. I'm only 11!

> Tommy: And I'm only nine! I'll see them win loads!

I reckon that's something that Chris, Grampy and Great-Granny Jen would be proud to hear. Howay the Toon.